THE
COMPLETE
FOOT BOOK

THE
COMPLETE
FOOT BOOK

Dr. Donald S. Pritt
Dr. Morton Walker

A DR. MORTON WALKER HEALTH BOOK

AVERY PUBLISHING GROUP INC.
Garden City Park, New York

This book has been written and published strictly for informational purposes. In no way should it be used as a substitute for your own health professional's advice. People who can make use of podiatric services should do so, for no amount of self-care is as good as the attention furnished by a trained, skilled, and knowledgeable doctor of podiatric medicine.

Cover Design: Ron Rodrigo
In-House Editor: Arthur Vidro
Typesetting: Widget Design; Mount Marion, New York
Original Artwork: Widget Design; Mount Marion, New York

Library of Congress Cataloging-in-Publication Data

Pritt, Donald S.
    The complete foot book : first aid for your feet / Donald S.
Pritt, Morton Walker.
      p. cm.
    Includes index.
    ISBN 0-89529-434-6 (pbk.)
    1. Foot—Care hygiene.   I. Walker, Morton.   II. Title.
    [DNLM: 1. Foot Diseases—popular works.   WE 880 P961c]
RD563P75 1992
617.5'85—dc20
DNLM/DLC
for Library of Congress   91-33326
                                                             CIP

Printed in the United States of America

10 9 8 7 6 5 4 3 2 1

Contents

To
Donald S. Pritt Jr.
and
Thomas S. Pritt

and to

Erica Walker
and
Jessica Walker

Preface

THE feet literally are the foundations of the body. They are the platform upon which the total body weight rests when a person stands, walks, runs, skips, or climbs. No building or any other kind of structure can long support itself if its foundations are weak or inadequate.

Yet, no part of the human body is as neglected as the foot. Although the feet are in almost constant use, we often take them for granted and pay little attention to their needs. That is, we ignore our feet until they give us trouble. So much are their well-being and comfort disregarded that perfect feet are rare.

While there is abundant literature for the foot specialist, little information on the foot exists for the average consumer. That is why a factual book dedicated to foot comfort has been urgently needed.

The Complete Foot Book goes beyond basic information and presents a variety of simple self-help, home-care techniques that every person can use for personal foot comfort and better foot health in general. The book is meant for people who want feet that don't hurt or who just want to learn more about their feet.

Weak feet, often inherited, are a part of being human, especially in a technological society.

The feet use a leverage principle to move body weight when walking, running, skipping, or performing other movements. Long toes, like a monkey's, would have hampered such motion and altered the leverage; consequently, evolutionary changes have caused human toes to become small and relatively stunted. But such stunting leaves the toes vulnerable to malformation, especially when their 'delicate structures are compressed by footgear that doesn't in any way resemble the shape of the feet.

The arch of each foot comprises twenty-six bones fitted together to work smoothly in unison. Unfortunately, arches sometimes become weakened to the point of collapse. The occurrence of so-called "fallen arches" is part of the human inheritance.

Foot problems should not develop if the muscles remain in tone, the ligaments stay firm, the bones retain their strength, and other foot tissues remain viable. But those deteriorations do occur, and mankind is more prone to the pain and problems of foot ill-health than to any other type of mechanical body failure. Indeed, foot and back problems equally cause discomfort for people in industrialized nations.

The result? Almost ninety percent of the 250 million people in the United States will, at one time or another in their lives, seek assistance for some type of foot ailment. It's then that people look for professional help; buy drugstore remedies, special molded footgear, orthopedic shoes, or arch supports; or try some other means of ridding themselves of the discomfort. It's a sad tale of miserable pain in the lower limbs.

The profession of podiatric medicine—foot doctoring—has attempted to help victims who suffer from the pain of ingrown toenails, bunions, dropped metatarsals, hammertoes, hard corns, soft corns, nerve corns, seed corns, calluses, plantar warts, fungus infections, and other foot miseries. Podiatrists sometimes don't come up with solutions for the multiple maladies that strike people. That's why a book describing what you can do to help yourself has become necessary.

The podiatry profession has been carrying on its battle against foot disabilities since 1912. Since then, the feet of North Americans, Europeans, Asians, Africans, and others have received preventive care against, protection from, and correction of painful problems. Doctors of podiatric medicine have tried their best to adapt whatever modern techniques they could from medicine, dentistry, and the other healing professions. They have developed their own methods, too. And a specialty branch of podiatrists has arisen: the Academy of Ambulatory Foot Surgeons.

These specialists keep you walking, running, skipping, and moving along with ease by using a dramatic new series of methods to correct the foot troubles besetting most of the world's industrialized countries. New surgical methods that entail minimal incisions correct foot deformities that once would have required large skin openings. The new methods have greatly reduced the chances for surgical side effects such as pain and bacterial infection. A person whose foot problems have been corrected with minimal-incision surgery can leave the doctor's office under his or her own power. Hospitals are no longer necessary for such procedures. Seldom is bed confinement required. On the contrary, the patient often returns to work immediately. Ambulatory foot surgery is not traumatic, particularly if mild painkillers are taken, and it usually requires very little convalescence time.

Ambulatory foot surgery corrects existing foot problems, but it's also used by podiatrists to protect against more serious maladies. Minimal incisions performed skillfully can protect people from those inherited foot weaknesses waiting to hamstring them into disability.

Let's face it. Nobody needs or wants foot trouble. Now that there is a comfortable way to solve those problems permanently, no one has to ignore or endure painful, persistent foot conditions.

The Complete Foot Book suggests easy, inexpensive ways to overcome your own foot problems by using whatever items are at hand, whether you are in your office, at home, at the factory, on vacation, or even in your automobile. This book guides you to total foot ease. But in case you are not quite able to achieve the comfortable result that you desire, a description of how ambulatory foot surgery can accomplish permanent correction of your difficulty is included at the end of many chapters.

Our aim as doctors of podiatric medicine — until recently, one was in a foot health care practice on a full-time basis; the other left podiatric surgery more than twenty-two years ago to work as a medical journalist — is to instruct you in how to find foot comfort for the rest of your lives. We wish you the ongoing ability to walk and be healthy.

Donald S. Pritt
Doctor of Podiatric Medicine
Vienna, West Virginia

Morton Walker
Doctor of Podiatric Medicine
Stamford, Connecticut

Part One

Foot Care, Footwear, and Foot Repair

1. *The Fabulous Human Foot*

THE structure of the human foot—your foot—is a fabulous piece of engineering design. Like an arched bridge that supports a great weight, it is highly functional and carries a tremendous load of pressure and pounds.

Your foot is an intricate mechanism. When commanded, it lifts and marches, turns and bends, and even kicks or shuffles. By a complex interworking of bones, muscles, nerves, blood vessels, and connective tissues, all concealed beneath the skin and nails, your feet propel your body in an amazing variety of movements, endure the weight of your body and the garments you wear, and stand up to the physical stresses involved. The efficiency and grace of nearly every movement of your body is related to the soundness of the supporting foundation provided by your feet.

Whether a human being has large or small feet, is tall or short, fat or thin, there are twenty-eight bones (including two tiny sesamoids) in each foot. The bones form four arches, are held together by 112 ligaments, and are activated by twenty muscles. Networks of blood vessels and nerves serve both the skeletal and the muscular structures of the foot.

Knowledge of the foot's different parts is essential in understanding its function, proper care, and ailments. Only when you understand the amazing engineering design within your feet can you appreciate the care that must be given them, not merely when they hurt, but every day. This first chapter, therefore, is devoted to describing the foot's structure and how it works.

BONES OF THE FOOT

The twenty-eight bones in each foot divide naturally into three groups. At the front of the foot are the fourteen *phalanges* that constitute the toes. In the middle of the foot are the five metatarsal and two sesamoid bones that together make up the *metatarsus,* or instep. At the back of the foot are the seven bones that form the *tarsus,* or heel and ankle: three wedge-shaped cuneiform bones; a boat-shaped navicular bone; a cube-shaped cuboid bone; the talus, or anklebone; and the calcaneus, or heel bone. (Figure 1.1 shows where the bones are located and how they join together.)

The main bone of the foot is the calcaneus, or heel bone. The talus, or anklebone, rests directly upon it. The weight of the body is transmitted through the anklebone downward to the other bones of the foot. Part of the weight is distributed downward and backward to the heel bone, and part is distributed downward and forward to the navicular.

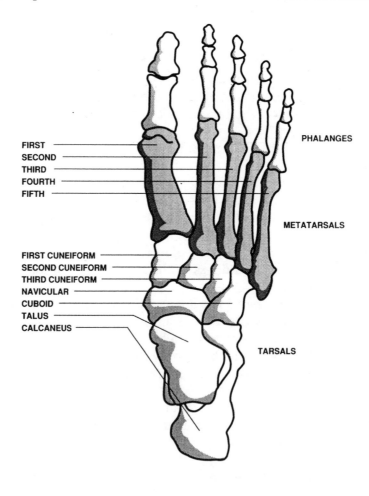

FIRST
SECOND
THIRD
FOURTH
FIFTH

PHALANGES

METATARSALS

FIRST CUNEIFORM
SECOND CUNEIFORM
THIRD CUNEIFORM
NAVICULAR
CUBOID
TALUS
CALCANEUS

TARSALS

Figure 1.1
The skeleton of the foot is an engineering marvel of twenty-eight bones and four arches. In this drawing, the foot's bones are viewed from above. Two sesamoid bones, located just beneath the first metatarsal bone, are not shown.

The navicular transmits weight to the three cuneiform bones, with which it joins. In turn, the three cuneiform bones join with and transmit weight to the first three metatarsal bones.

The cuboid, which is next to the navicular, receives the weight transmitted forward by the calcaneus and transmits it to the fourth and fifth metatarsal bones.

The five metatarsal bones, arranged on different planes, transmit weight to the forward part of the foot. Two small bones that are actually independent of the skeleton of the body, since they do not join with any other bones, are located under the head of the first metatarsal bone. They are known as sesamoid bones because they are shaped like sesame seeds. They float in the tendon of a small foot muscle and act to protect the tendon as it moves back and forth.

The phalanges of the toes join with the metatarsals. Each of the four small toes has three toe bones, but the big toe has only two. The toe bones, except for those of the big toe, bear almost no weight when you walk. Their principal function is to give spring to the step.

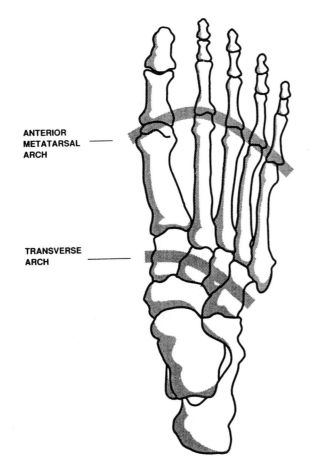

ANTERIOR
METATARSAL
ARCH

TRANSVERSE
ARCH

Figure 1.2
The anterior metatarsal arch and the transverse arch are clearly seen in this drawing of the top of the foot.

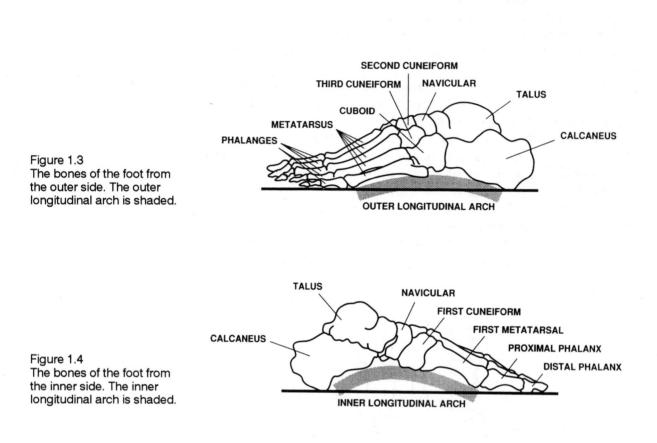

Figure 1.3
The bones of the foot from the outer side. The outer longitudinal arch is shaded.

Figure 1.4
The bones of the foot from the inner side. The inner longitudinal arch is shaded.

FOUR ARCHES OF THE FOOT

When the body is erect, its weight is transmitted through the anklebone to the other bones of the foot and is shared with them. The twenty-eight bones in the foot are so placed that they catch and bear the entire weight of the body on four arches. Two run across the foot; the other two run the length of the foot. (See Figures 1.2, 1.3, and 1.4.)

The *transverse arch*, which is formed by the three cuneiform bones and the cuboid, accepts your weight as it comes down the leg through the heel bone.

The *anterior metatarsal arch* is formed, at the point where the metatarsal bones join the phalanges, by the arrangement of the metatarsals on different planes—the first and fifth metatarsals are on a low plane; the second, third, and fourth are on higher planes. Because the metatarsals are free of muscle attachments, the foot is able to adjust to uneven ground. The anterior metatarsal arch flattens out when the front ends (the heads) of the metatarsals bear the weight.

The *outer longitudinal arch*, which is formed by the calcaneus, the cuboid, and the fourth and fifth metatarsals, is solid and flat. It receives and carries the major portion of the body's weight.

The *inner longitudinal arch*, which is formed by the calcaneus, the talus, the cuneiforms, and the three inner metatarsals, acts like a spring. It absorbs the natural shocks that come from walking.

FOOT JOINTS

The joints, or articulations, of the foot come in two types. The ankle and the toe joints are typical hinge articulations; that is, the hinge joint allows the ankle and toes to flex and bend up and down and to move forward and backward.

The other joints of the foot, those between tarsal bones or between the tarsal and metatarsal bones, are of a gliding nature, one against another. The tarsal and metatarsal bones can move only slightly — except for the ankle, which enjoys greater movement.

All the joints of the foot are protected by a covering of cartilage and are lubricated by synovial fluid. Ligaments of tough elastic fiber connect the bones one to another. A capsule surrounds each articulation and protects the delicate structures within.

FOOT AND LEG MUSCLES

Your foot cannot function without its twenty muscles and the muscles of the lower leg. They bend or extend the toes at the joints, raise or lower the toes singly or in groups, flex the sole of the foot, and in general make possible the great variety of movements or combinations of movements of the foot.

Nearly every foot movement involves some use of the leg muscles. Leg muscles raise your foot to a tiptoe position, rotate the foot, flex the ankle. The leg muscles balance the leg on the foot by alternately tensing and relaxing first one muscle group and then another. The balancing action causes the body weight to be carried on the strongest structures of the foot — the heel bone, the anklebone, and the first metatarsal. The leg muscles also counterbalance the forces that develop when the body is thrown off balance; for example, when you trip as you walk, those muscles act to restore your balance.

Some foot and leg muscles are matched in pairs: as one stretches, the other contracts. In such cases, long muscles are attached at one end to a bone in the leg and at the other end to a bone in the foot. In most cases, the leg muscle ends in a long tendon that extends through the foot to its point of attachment to the bone.

Working together in a coordinated effort to carry out the commands of the body, leg and foot muscles make possible such activities as standing, walking, running, jumping, and dancing.

TENDONS OF THE LOWER LIMB

Muscles end in tendons, fibrous cords of connective tissue that attach muscle to bone. A tendon is surrounded by a sheath of protective material that, in turn, is protected by layers of additional tough fibrous tissue. The Achilles tendon probably is the one best known; it runs from the middle of the back of the leg to the heel bone.

On the bottom of the foot are two groups of fibrous tissue called fasciae. Both those fasciae, long and slim but strong and tight as a bowstring, run from the heel to the toes, with slips of tissue extending into each toe. The fasciae help the inner and outer longitudinal arches absorb shocks to the foot and bear the stress that is caused by the body's weight.

BLOOD VESSELS OF THE FOOT

The foot's blood vessels form an extremely fine network of arteries, veins, and capillaries to provide the lowest extremity with a rich supply of blood, which carries nutrients to the cells.

The dorsalis pedis artery supplies fresh blood to the top of the foot. It is a continuation of the anterior tibial artery, which runs down the thigh and over the front of the leg. To locate the anterior tibial artery, place your fingers on the top of the foot over the first metatarsal at the instep—that is, on the top part of the foot in front of the ankle. You will feel a definite pulse, similar to the pulse in your wrist.

The posterior tibial artery supplies blood to the bottom of the foot. It runs down the back of the leg and around the anklebone, where it separates into several smaller branches. You can feel the pulse in this artery behind the anklebone on the inner side of the foot near the midline of the body.

Both the dorsalis pedis and the posterior tibial arteries branch out into arterioles, which subdivide into a network of minute arteries, or capillaries. The capillaries are so numerous that a compression bandage held tightly about the foot would not cut off all the blood that flows through them.

The veins that return the blood from the foot to the upper portions of the body run directly alongside the arteries. The dorsal and plantar metatarsal veins join with the saphenous vein to return blood to the

FOOT FACT

Nobody's feet are perfect. No person has two feet that totally match. And nobody's feet are exactly like anybody else's.

heart. Other veins of the foot connect with the front and back tibial veins.

NERVES THAT AFFECT THE FOOT

Like the blood vessels that serve the foot, the nerves follow a definite pattern. There are nerves that serve the bottom of the foot and nerves that innervate, or stimulate, the top; there are deep nerves and nerves for the skin.

The main nerves of the foot are continuations of the tibial and peroneal nerves, which stem from the lumbar and sacral regions of the spine and extend the entire length of the leg. Because of the patterns of those nerves, foot doctors can administer anesthetics above the foot. If, for example, a local anesthetic is injected at specific places in the ankle, then large areas on the sole of the foot will lose sensitivity.

THE FOOT'S COVERING

The skin of the foot is of two types, described simply as thick skin and thin skin. The sole of the foot is composed entirely of thickened skin, which can be up to five layers deep. (Most areas of the body contain only one layer of skin.) Thick skin has no hair follicles or oil glands. When prolonged pressure or friction is applied to thick skin, the outermost layer grows into a leathery, horny mass that we call a callus. Thick skin on the foot forms a mat tough enough to protect the weight-bearing bones from injury. The thick skin of the sole also protects the many structures inside the foot against abrasions, lacerations, and perforations by sharp objects. The ridges and whorls on the foot's thick skin, very much like those that appear in fingerprints, give rise to friction and thus supply a grasping surface for the bare foot.

Thin skin is the normal epidermis. Thin skin covers the whole foot except for the sole and toenails. Like the thin skin on the rest of the body, it consists of only one layer, which contains oil glands and hair follicles.

FOOT FACT

Toenails and fingernails grow fastest in hot weather, in pregnancy, and during the teen years. Their rate of growth is inherited; there's nothing you can do to speed it up.

TOENAILS THAT PROTECT

Toenails are the familiar, hard, horny, colorless, little protective plates that cover the top end of each toe. A toenail emerges from a growth center, or nail root, that is implanted a short distance behind the visible portion of the nail in a groove in the skin. The exposed, translucent portion of the toenail is the nail body, or nail plate. (See Figure 1.5.) The free end is called the free margin. The part of the nail that is out of sight between the body and the root is known as the matrix. At the base of the nail, where it appears at the edge of the skin fold, the nail does not adhere to the flesh; there, a white, half-moon portion called the lunula appears.

Skin covers a narrow margin of the back of the nail near the matrix to form the cuticle. At each side of the nail is a fleshy fold that partially covers the edge. Beneath the fleshy fold is a nail groove through which the nail rides as it grows outward. Underneath each toenail is a network of blood vessels and longitudinal ridges. It is the pinkish hue of those blood vessels that is visible through the translucent nail plate.

A toenail grows, usually in a straight line, from the nail root, not from the free end. Injury to the matrix or root interrupts the nail's natural protective growth pattern; the toenail would then grow either abnormally thick or to one side.

WHAT DO YOUR FEET DO?

Although you use your feet mostly for walking, they also support or carry your body when you are standing, running, climbing, descending, jumping, or doing special locomotion such as dancing.

When you walk, the foot acts as a lever. The muscles in the back of the leg pull up against gravity. Weight is transferred in rapid order from the anklebone to the heel bone, down the outer longitudinal arch, across the metatarsal heads, and off the big toe. Thus the body weight is propelled forward toward the ball of the foot (the area where the metatarsal heads touch the ground). The center of gravity of the body

Figure 1.5
This cross section depicts the anatomy of a toenail. It is an avascular structure but has some nerve sensitivity, which is protected underneath by thickened skin.

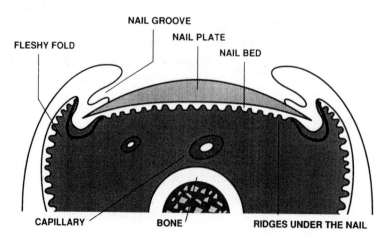

is shifted to a few inches in front of the toes at a point not yet occupied by the person. At the same time, the other foot is moved forward by the thigh and hip. The muscles in the front of the leg contract the inner longitudinal arch and prepare it to accept the weight of the body as the heel comes down in a forward motion. The muscles in the feet themselves raise the arch and act as a spring that helps support the inner longitudinal arch and increase the stability of the foot.

That complicated group of movements requires a coordination of the body's muscles as a whole. Many of those movements are controlled by reflexes. For instance, walking is a continuous process of losing and regaining balance. Although walking is a voluntary movement, a baby needs continual practice to develop the reflexes into automatic movements that thereafter will be under the control of the higher brain centers.

Standing involves transmitting the weight from the anklebone to the heel bone to the ground. The other structures provide only balance.

Running is locomotion in which the weight of the body is transmitted only to the front of the foot; that is, the toes and ball of the foot alone touch the ground. In some kinds of running, both feet occasionally are off the ground at the same time. Because running throws the body's center of gravity far forward, the foot, as it comes down to make contact with the ground, is actually catching the full weight of the body.

Climbing—for example, ascending stairs—requires actual physical force to lift the weight of the body from the heel onto the front of the foot. Descending stairs places the weight of your body on the front of the foot, where it is held until the heel comes into contact with the step. The weight and increased pressure of gravity as you descend is then carried along the entire sole of the foot until the other foot comes forward to bear the weight.

Jumping requires lifting both feet off the ground at the same time. Just before the jump, a great deal of strain is placed on the foot in bringing together a coordinated muscular action. The ligaments play a major role in producing a spring with an interaction of all the joints.

Ballroom dancing requires the weight to be carried on the front portion of the foot in a rhythmic motion. Reflex action comes into play to produce smooth and gliding movement.

The human foot, as you can see, is a marvel of coordinated action and effort by each part of its structure. There is nothing else quite like it in the world. It is as distinctively human as the trunk is elephantine. The foot allows man to walk upright in a way that no other animal can quite imitate; and it carries out its locomotive functions with vigor, efficiency, and grace. Indeed, the foot has been a major factor in mankind's mastery of Earth.

FOOT FACT

Runners hit the ground with a force two and a half times their body weight.

2. *Basic Foot Care*

To anthropologists, it's no surprise that men, women, and even children commonly suffer from foot trouble. The cause goes back to the beginning of mankind when ape-like creatures who had walked on all fours rose to the bipedal position. Each foot had once carried twenty-five percent of the body's weight but now was burdened with fifty percent. Furthermore, feet today are subjected to more stress as a result of walking on flat, unyielding pavements, hardwood floors, concrete, asphalt, tile, steel, and other unnatural ground coverings. This change has brought its own particular set of difficulties.

Muscle wastage has appeared in human lower extremities during the past hundred years, primarily because of a lack of exercise. Modern transportation conveniences in our society have led to the feet and legs being used less today than they were when people depended more on walking to get from place to place.

As individuals become older, particular foot problems develop. Anthropologists are not surprised, and neither are foot doctors. They know that most people possess one of the three types of feet that cause pain and other problems.

Each foot contains a set of twenty-eight bones, but foot typing comes only from the thickness, shape, and length of a person's toes. Checking your feet against the following descriptions will let you know if you have one of the three types of problem-causing feet.

MUSICAL FOOT

First is the exceedingly wide foot having splayed bones that get squeezed together by footgear. We call the type with such an accordion compression the "musical foot" because it plays a painful tune for its victim. His or her foot bones are rather flexible, as if held together by a bag of skin.

In the musical foot, wide spaces exist between each of the five long metatarsal bones. The big toe bends toward the midline of the body; the little toe bends outward. You'll most likely see a bunion on the inner (big toe) side of the foot and a bulbous knob on the outer (fifth toe) side. Plus, there probably will be a dropped metatarsal arch, which usually carries a thickness of callus on the bottom of the foot. The burning callus smarts with each step. Corns might be present on the edges of the first and fifth toes. The corns hurt terribly in most instances and can even incapacitate the person. Walking is miserable for the person with such fan-shaped feet, causing him or her to sing a song of woe.

BUNIONED FOOT

Some feet have long first toes accompanied by red, hot, swollen, and sometimes painful bunion joints. Such joints arise from two sources: an inherent weakness within the big toe joint, and counterpressure by the shoe as it butts back against the toe tip with each step forward. Such force pushes the big toe into an angle that causes a bunion to pop out and eventually to become permanent as a result of calcification of soft tissues.

The bunion is simply an irritation at first. But it rubs itself so much that body fluid finally engorges the tissues. Stockings that fit too tightly can further compound the problem. Eventually the fluid formed around the bunion inflammation solidifies and turns into calcium deposits. A hard and bony bunion called a *hallux valgus* results, and surgery is often needed to eliminate it. Pain is ever present for the sufferer with a bunioned foot.

MORTON'S SYNDROME FOOT

The third type of foot usually susceptible to problems has long second toes and short first toes. In 1935, Dr. Dudley J. Morton, professor of anatomy at the College of Physicians and Surgeons of Columbia University, described those feet. The foot type has since been named Morton's syndrome foot.

A Morton's syndrome foot usually has painful calluses under the front part of the enlarged second metatarsal. The calluses invariably thicken to the point that central nuclei form underneath the foot at the prominence of the metatarsal heads. The skin burns with each step taken. Also, the second, third, or fourth toes often experience hammering. With hammertoe, one or more toes overlap adjacent toes; corns develop on the areas formed by the overlapping bones. A Morton's syndrome foot requires attention if its owner is to find comfort.

QUESTIONS TO ASK YOURSELF

Do you possess one of the three types of problem feet? Which one? Most of the foot troubles that beset adults come from one of those three foot types.

Are your feet widespread bags of bones with knobs on both sides and calluses underneath? Do you have long first toes with painful bunions? Do you have shortened big toes with extended second toes, second metatarsal calluses under your feet, and hammertoes? Over eighty-five percent of all people who wear leather shoes have one of those foot types.

Whether you find the descriptions funny, shocking, or repulsive, such conditions bring no pleasure to their owners. Problem foot types produce tears of pain in the eyes of their possessors. Yet relief is available; no one needs to suffer. You only have to recognize the foot type you have and take self-help or professional corrective measures to cope.

BASIC CARE FOR THE FEET

No vaccine or pill can prevent disorders of the feet, but specific health habits can spare you foot trouble. Still, many persons are unaware of the existence of preventive foot health. It is difficult to convince a child, a teenager, or even an adult that he will have foot trouble later in life if he fails to care for his feet now. Yet, current statistics indicate that unless the public is educated in habits of good foot care, most people will suffer from foot problems as they age.

You can help yourself. Probably more than eighty percent of our foot ills are self-inflicted; of those, ninety-five percent can be prevented. Some podiatrists assert that of the approximately five hundred different foot ailments, the majority arise from improper foot care. If we would devote to foot health the amount of time we spend in brushing our teeth, we could practically assure ourselves of lifelong foot comfort and spare ourselves the inconvenience, expense, and pain that foot neglect always brings.

FOOT FACT

More women than men develop blisters, corns, bunions, calluses, ingrown toenails, and cold feet. More men than women have athlete's foot, foot injuries, and malodorous feet.

What to Look for When Purchasing Hosiery

The two main functions of stockings, socks, and other forms of hosiery are to absorb moisture from the feet and to protect them against irritation from rubs, cracks in the shoe's leather, and other potential sources of friction.

Socks should be about a half-inch longer than the foot, should give the toes room to wiggle, and generally should fit smoothly snug but not too tight. Socks should not produce folds or wrinkles, and they should not have any seams: those are all causes of irritation.

Fitted socks are better than tube socks for exact fit, but tube socks last longer because you don't wear out the same spots with repeated usage. Natural fibers—cotton and wool—have a greater ability to absorb moisture than do acrylic fibers. Bicyclists and soccer players usually find that thin socks give them more of a barefoot feel, while tennis and basketball players prefer hosiery with more bulk and padding for greater shock absorption.

Some of the newer stockings have high-density padding at key stress points on the footed portion to provide extra protection during vigorous activity.

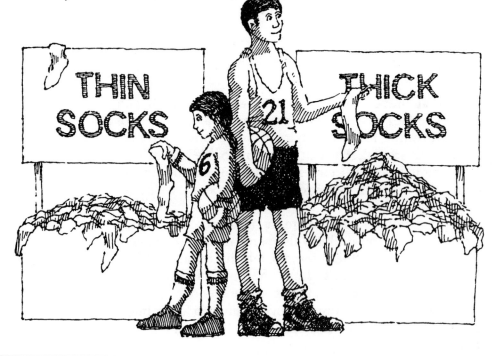

Just a handful of do's and don'ts—if followed diligently—can save you from hours of discomfort and spare you more serious difficulties. The following sets of rules are basic, even elementary, but people too often ignore these simplest of practices that would prevent foot discomfort.

EIGHT ACTIONS TO GET HAPPY FEET

Observe these eight simple rules for everyday foot care and avoid the majority of painful foot ailments:

- Wash your feet daily with soap and warm water, using a washcloth or soapy fingers to clean between the toes. This rule hardly is sophisticated advice, but it sometimes is totally neglected, especially by elderly people, who tend to pay less attention to their personal hygiene, and by children, who of course must always be supervised.
- After bathing, dry the feet well—completely dry!—with a rough terry-cloth towel. Remember that moisture between the toes is a major cause of athlete's foot.
- Rub lubricating cream into any dry, scaly skin on the heels or toes. The cream you use on your hands or face is also good for your feet. Your podiatrist will prescribe a cream if you request it.
- Dust your feet, if they sweat profusely, with foot powder containing an anti-fungal ingredient. Even if your feet do not perspire, shake some powder into your shoes every morning.
- Wear shoes a quarter-inch wider, and socks or stockings half to three-quarters of an inch longer, than the foot. Allowing enough room in shoes and stockings to wiggle your toes may prevent a deformity.
- Change your hose and shoes frequently. Keep your shoes in good repair. You should have at least two pairs of shoes that you can alternate daily; accumulated perspiration must be allowed to dry out. A fresh pair of socks should be worn every day; if you perspire excessively, switch to a second pair during the day.
- Clip your toenails straight across with a standard toenail clipper. Square corners prevent ingrown nails. To facilitate the clipping of dry, brittle nails, soften them first by soaking them in warm, soapy water.
- When walking or standing, hold yourself erect with your weight distributed evenly on both feet.

(The exercises illustrated in chapter twenty offer additional ways to help your feet.)

EIGHT PODIATRIC PITFALLS

Observe these eight simple rules of what not to do if you want to avoid complications in your foot health:

FOOT FACT

Though it sounds
uncomfortable, a few
runners trot along
barefoot. Perhaps the
most famous was
distance runner Zola
Budd, who won several
races barefoot in the
early 1980s.

- Do not use foot remedies that can cause chemical burns, inflammations, infections, or general sepsis. Overtreatment of a condition can cause damage under the skin to tender tissues, which may not have lines of defense against fungal, viral, or bacterial invasion. Keep in mind that patented preparations sold over the counter, while useful in many instances, are not likely to offer permanent eradication of athlete's foot or other skin conditions. It is best to get professional advice from your doctor, in particular from a podiatrist, who specializes in taking care of foot problems. Other times, an orthopedic surgeon or your family's general practitioner may help.
- Although corn cures, iodine, toenail outgrow, and other commercial products may temporarily alleviate foot pain, those items often tend to aggravate the initial condition. Therefore, do not rely solely on drugstore remedies as your source of foot health. Certainly don't try such cures at random. Ask your friendly local podiatrist instead; he or she can advise you on your specific difficulty.
- Do not unnecessarily expose your feet and legs to dampness and cold. Those environmental conditions not only interfere with blood circulation, but they may be a contributing cause of osteoarthritis and other degenerative diseases.
- Do not overuse hot-water bottles or electric heating pads. If you must apply them to feet for purposes of warmth, then make certain they are not so hot that they burn the skin. Such devices might also cause blood circulatory problems later on.
- Do not cut your corns and calluses with dull or dirty instruments. Instead, use sharp razor blades or scissors, but only after they've been sterilized in boiling water. Dull tools make for bleeding that is difficult to control. Dirty instruments might bring on an infection.
- Do not sit with your knees crossed for long periods, and don't wear circular garters or constrictive bandages. Doing so risks cutting off the blood to your legs and toes.
- Never wear another person's shoes or slippers. The fungi that cause athlete's foot live in shoes; infected shoes can transmit the disease to anyone who wears them.
- Never walk barefoot on concrete pavement, asphalt, or tile or hardwood floors. Walking barefoot is allowable only on beach sand, lawns, carpeting, and other pliable materials.

Perhaps you have often thought of those do's and don'ts. But if you want to enjoy better foot health, then make them part of your daily routine.

Anytime you take a tool to the skin of your feet, you are opening yourself to potential difficulties. The feet are not the cleanest part of the human body. Whether in shoes or bare, they have to walk about in the polluted environment that humans have created. Wearing shoes does not protect our feet totally, for microorganisms can lodge in our footgear.

Nevertheless, the modern generation often wears shoes without a protective layer of hosiery. Such action, although lately fashionable, is downright unhealthy. The non-wearing of socks or stockings is a pet peeve of health professionals.

The best hosiery for you has full cotton or wool at the foot portion. Avoid hosiery containing polyester or other plastic fibers. But for your feet's sake, wear hosiery.

3. *Are You Breaking in Your Shoes or Your Feet?*

IT might surprise you to learn that the feet of a man who weighs 178 pounds lift about 3.2 million pounds every day just by carrying him around. Is it any wonder that many of us come to the end of a long, hard day of labor, sports participation, or shopping groaning that our feet hurt?

Of course, persons enjoying excellent health who also have feet that are in perfect, or nearly perfect, condition do not normally suffer from tired feet every day. Yet even the strongest and healthiest individuals are acquainted with some degree of foot fatigue.

The 3.2 million-pound figure is based on statistics provided by the United States Department of Labor. To compute the approximate burden that your feet carry each day, multiply your body weight by the number of steps—18,000 of them—that the average person takes daily. At a rate of 18,000 steps a day, the average person walks one thousand miles a year! Can you imagine taking an automobile trip of such a length on anything less than well-maintained tires?

Isn't it just as reasonable to insist that the condition of your feet is important to health and comfort? That your feet deserve every effort to keep them fit and healthy?

HOW TO CHOOSE FOOTGEAR

Everyone does not perform the same kind of work, so the same demands are not made of everyone's feet. If you labor in a lumberyard

FOOT FACT

The ancient Romans were the first to create distinct left and right shoes; previously, all shoes could be worn on either foot.

21

and carry planks all day, your feet will be subjected to more physical demands than if you sit and do bookkeeping. However, the individual at a desk will not necessarily have better feet than the worker who stands or trudges all day. Regardless of a person's job, feet encased in poorly built, ill-fitted, or badly run-down shoes will be subjected hour after hour and day after day to harsh treatment.

What type of shoes should you wear at work? The answer, of course, depends upon the work you do. A farmer or forester who stomps along on rough, uneven terrain will want a high shoe or boot that supports the ankle. A clerk or salesperson in a department store might prefer a low shoe such as a pump, a loafer, or an oxford.

The oxford, in its various forms, is the most popular shoe today and the most supportive all-purpose form of footwear. For the majority of people, the oxford is perfectly satisfactory to wear at work. But any shoe that has the same essential features as the oxford can be a comfortable work shoe. Such a shoe should have a thick, hard sole made of leather, rubber, or composition; a broad heel less than two inches high; and a steel shank. (The shank, which lies between the insole and the outsole, acts as a shock absorber between the foot and the ground.) Finally, it must possess an external fastening—laces, buckles, or straps—to hold it securely on the foot. A shoe with those features will protect the foot and, if it fits properly, will do the most to ensure foot health while you are at work.

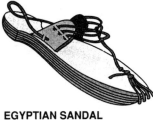

**EGYPTIAN SANDAL
AGE OF THE PHARAOHS**

How the shoes fit, their condition, and their appropriateness to the tasks you perform all affect your feet by the end of the day. The wrong shoe can, of course, cause you pain, but the effects of wearing an incorrect shoe can reach much further.

Incorrect footgear is likely to reduce your job efficiency. The Women's Bureau of the United States Department of Labor states, "The shoes women wear at work have a greater effect on their comfort, safety, and efficiency than any other item of clothing." For example, party shoes, casual shoes, and worn-out shoes have no place in the factory, store, field, forest, or office. They lead only to foot and leg fatigue. And high heels—heels in excess of two inches—have no place on a woman's foot whether she is cooking, food shopping, cleaning, walking a distance, addressing a jury, or making the rounds on a hospital ward.

The task of choosing a pair of shoes is, or at least should be, more than a minor chore to be hurried through during a lunch break. Many persons, men and women alike, ignore what should be a simple matter of common sense—that the selection of a pair of shoes to be worn over many months, a year, or longer deserves at least as much care as the buying of a hat. But too many shoppers approach the task knowing little or nothing about foot function or shoe construction and end up selecting shoes either from habit or simply to be in fashion. No wonder they ultimately suffer from uncomfortable or ailing feet.

SHOE STYLES

The most common, popular, and supportive shoe style for decades has been the oxford, which is worn by men, women, and children. However modified or decorated, it remains the same in its essentials: it is laced; it has a low, broad heel and a more or less rounded toe; and its upper rises only as far as the top of the heel.

The safety shoe is a variation on the oxford (although a boot can also be a safety shoe). It has a sturdy leather upper, a roomy toe, and steel or otherwise reinforced toe caps that guard against crushing from heavy items dropped onto the foot. It has saved thousands of workers from injurious, even crippling, accidents. Its insulated, suction-like, rubber, corded soles offer protection on greasy or hot floors. There have been many adaptations of the safety shoe to fit different circumstances. One variation that protects the toes and is often used after foot surgery uses a covering of wire mesh to create a sort of cage effect.

Loafers, sneakers, running shoes, beach shoes, and sandals have their places in casual everyday wear—for lounging at the poolside, attending a lawn party, boating, or resting at home. However, in the business world, where one must walk on hard, flat, tiled floors or on the concrete pavement of city streets, those shoe types are less desirable.

The loafer is probably one of the major causes of corns on the tops of toes. The stitching on a loafer permits the leather to stretch, so the shoe tends to become larger and sloppy with wear. It stays on the foot only because the wearer contracts his toes, thus broadening his metatarsal area and expanding his foot in the shoe. The friction of a loafer's rubbing against the contracted toes leads to the forming of corns. External fastenings on the shoes can prevent that effect. Indeed, the lack of fastenings on any shoe is a serious disadvantage in terms of foot health.

Shoes with cleats offer greater traction and are used in track, baseball, football, golf, and other sports. Although the cleats certainly are useful, they can be a source of irritation, for much of the weight is carried on the small areas of the shoe sole where the cleats are attached.

Ski boots, ice skates, and bowling shoes must fit snugly in the longitudinal arches if they are to give proper balance and support. A snug fit is especially important in ski boots, for the danger of breaking a bone while skiing is always present. Similarly, ice skates should fit snugly to prevent muscles from tightening, which could lead to acutely painful spasms.

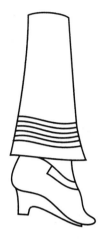

**CHINESE GIRL'S
BOUND FOOT**

THE ART OF SHOEMAKING

Shoemaking is a gentle craft—or so legend has it. Two early Christian martyrs, the brothers Crispin and Crispinian, are the patron saints of

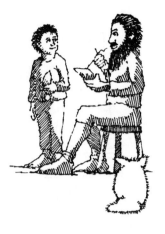

shoemakers. Until they were killed for their religious beliefs by the Romans in about the year 280, those gentle cobblers, like Robin Hoods of the foot care world, stole leather to make shoes for the poor. While they stitched shoes, they spread the word of Christianity.

But there is nothing gentle about the shoemaking process today. Except in the making of high-quality custom shoes and in the repairing of shoes, the artisan of yesteryear has been supplanted by machines. Leather-sewing machines, automatic splitting machines, sole-cutting machines, and other devices have been perfected for use in almost every operation involved in the construction of footwear. As many as 170 distinct operations are performed in the manufacture of a single pair of shoes. The assembly-line method of construction means as many as 210 persons operate the machines that perform the various tasks.

Shoe materials have varied through the ages, but leather has always been regarded in highest favor. Leather is strong, durable, and not too expensive; leather also "breathes." The breathing property has been a point of controversy in the leather industry for years. Many question whether leather produced by modern methods can breathe after being subjected to so many chemical treatments during the tanning process; they contend that modern tanning must surely eliminate some of the air spaces and pores of the leather.

Other materials used for shoes include canvas, for sneakers; felt, for slippers; straw, for beach shoes; paper, for throwaways; rubber, for wearing in the shower or in the rain; and plastics of all types.

Synthetic materials are constantly being tested for footwear. However, many of them fail. For instance, Corfam, a plastic artificial leather developed and marketed in the 1960s, was scuffproof, needed no polishing, and was uniform in texture and thickness. Leather has none of those qualities. Yet, Corfam, which promised to revolutionize the shoe industry as nylon had revolutionized the stocking and clothing industries, turned out to be a bust. It was too heavy on the feet. When made into a pair of shoes, it weighed about three times more than leather and felt awfully heavy to walk around in. Corfam shoes brought on fatigue quickly. The result? Corfam enjoyed popularity for a dozen years and then faded out of existence.

SHOE QUALITY

Shoe quality is important. Fit, appropriateness, and quality of materials make the shoe right or wrong for you.

With the advent of new plastics and synthetics, soling materials in addition to leather, crepe, rubber, and sponge have become possible. Whatever the material, soles must be thick enough to resist the impact when the shoe strikes a hard object, such as a rock. When the ball of the foot strikes the ground, the sole should not be so flexible as to cave inward. Otherwise, too much weight will be placed suddenly on one metatarsal bone. The thin soles on a woman's high-heeled pumps or on a teenager's one-strap dancing flats are often too flexible when they strike a hard object.

What is even more important than the soling is the shank. Every good shoe should have a metal shank, preferably a piece of steel about three to five inches long and half an inch wide, within the sole of the shoe. The shank accepts the buffeting from walking or running and absorbs vibrations that otherwise would reverberate throughout the body. It gives quality to a well-made pair of shoes.

Be aware, too, that what the upper of the shoe is made of is not as important as how the shoe fits all over. The upper should not constrain or contort the feet, and there must be sufficient width and length to the whole shoe.

HISTORY OF FOOTWEAR

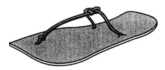

**SLAVE SANDAL
ABOUT 1300**

Almost from their beginning, humans have worn various sandals, clogs, boots, animal skin wrappings, and other shoe-like forms to protect their feet. Even before the arrival of what we call civilization, primitive man wore what may be called, for lack of a better word, shoes. Animal skins wrapped around his feet afforded the caveman some protection from rough, stony ground. Today, men and women continue to wrap animal skins around their feet, but the skins are dressed and tanned and styled in more elaborate fashion. Early man protected himself from the irregularity of the surfaces on which he walked, but today people most often wear shoes to protect themselves against the flatness, hardness, and smoothness of floors, pavements, and sidewalks.

Of all the items of footwear currently worn, the sandal is the simplest and probably the oldest. The Egyptians, Hebrews, Greeks, and Romans all wore sandals. Even today, the sandal is the major article of footwear in the Orient. It is, of course, quite popular for summerwear in the United States.

Today's sandal, unlike the shoe and the boot, has no solid upper covering. It is primarily a shoe with straps that buckle across the foot or lace around the ankle and lower leg. Sandals have changed over the years. The ancient Hebrews, for example, made theirs of leather, rawhide, cloth, felt, or wood and secured them to their feet with thongs or latches. The sandals of all the early civilizations were worn principally to protect the sole of the foot and not as articles of adornment.

Modern footwear was born during the late crusades, when feudalism was coming to an end and the Renaissance was dawning. During that period, both the boot and the shoe gradually developed.

The boot is footwear that extends above the ankle; it may reach as high as the knee or even cover part of the lower thigh. What distinguishes the boot from the shoe, the most familiar footgear today, is that a shoe extends only to the ankle and not above. Like a boot, a shoe may be buttoned, buckled, laced, or strapped, or it may have no external fastening.

Since the Renaissance, shoes in the Western world (except perhaps in the lands of the far north) have been shaped primarily for ornamental consideration rather than protective function. Precious jewels, big buckles of metal or ivory, satin ribbons, and the finest tapestries have all been used in an attempt to beautify the feet by adorning the shoes. The hazards of cold, moisture, and rough terrain have been disregarded, and the natural shape and function of the foot have been ignored, while the shoe has been fashioned in all sorts of bizarre shapes, variations, and styles. But because there has been one unalterable factor—the human foot itself—the basic design of shoes has remained largely unaltered.

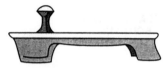

TURKISH SANDAL 1660

THOUGHTS ON MODERN SHOE DESIGN

Studies of the foot since the advent of modern medicine have taught us the dynamics of the foot in standing, running, jumping, climbing, and dancing. That knowledge enables us to design the proper shoe for the proper occasion. Contemporary shoe designers, unfortunately, seem to be perplexed by how the foot actually works. For they continue to produce outlandish, malfunctional fashions—especially for women. As a consequence, the modern woman's shoes do considerable damage to her feet.

The contemporary shoe designer, if one may judge by his or her creations, is convinced that the foot should fit the shoe rather than the other way around. Designers appear to insist that the shoe is primarily an object of fashion. By creating a beautiful object into which to put the foot, the shoe designer strives to make the foot beautiful. Still, few feet are truly beautiful. Besides, when a beautiful foot is shod in one of the contemporary designer's "beautiful" creations, and is kept there, it soon ceases to be beautiful. Designers have chosen to forget that the foot is made of flesh and blood, that it is only so pliable, and that to make unreasonable demands upon it serves only to destroy its comfort as well as its beauty.

Shoe designers constantly revive historical designs, and thus the old, malfunctional shoe fashions are repeated in cycles—with disastrous results. What can be done about it? Nothing, as long as the wearer does not demand shoes that fit well and take into account the work the feet must do. If women would refuse to buy footwear that causes them to suffer aches, pains, and foot trouble, then shoe designers would probably concentrate on creating more healthful fashions.

Already, some shoe manufacturers are providing a few styles that take foot anatomy into account. While the authors choose not to promote specific brand names, we acknowledge that designers have created a few new fashions that cause no crippling and still look attractive.

No matter what our intentions when we go to buy shoes, few of us ignore fashion completely. But neither should we ignore the fact that if we supinely buy shoes that will cause us foot abuse and discomfort, then we will have only ourselves to blame.

Why we behave so strangely when we buy footgear might make for an interesting psychological study. No one in his right mind would wear a hat that squeezed his head into the shape of a pyramid, yet an otherwise brilliant woman, shrewd in business, excellent as a housewife and mother, submits to the wearing of shoes that squeeze her feet into pointed pie-like wedges.

Psychologists have, in fact, verified that the modern woman has a need to be part of the crowd; that is why she follows the fashion styles wherever they lead. If fashion leaders raise the hemline this year, she might raise hers. If next year they lower the hemline, she might lower hers. And what is true for dress in general is just as true for shoes. (It must be noted that men are not free from this need to conform; they are less susceptible only because their garment styles change less frequently and less dramatically.)

Such behavior is not ordinarily dangerous. A new fashion in a skirt or blouse may be uncomfortable or unsuitable, but that generally is as far as it goes. Even such uncomfortable items as girdles and brassieres are worn year after year by millions of women without causing apparent harm.

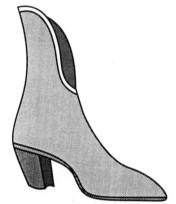

COLONIAL SHOE 1725

Shoes are another matter, however. Shoes can be not only uncomfortable but, in many instances, dangerous. Shoe fashions, therefore, affect not only the feet but the health of the individual.

HOW TO BUY SHOES WISELY

Incorrect footgear can do much harm to your body. Therefore, we have devised eight simple rules for buying shoes:

- Do not tell the salesperson your shoe size. Insist that he or she measure your feet. Your foot size might change between purchases. Since a half-size is only one-sixth of an inch, a very small change in the length of your foot can require your wearing a larger shoe.

- Make sure that the clerk measures both feet twice, once when you are standing and again when you are sitting.
- Make certain that the material of the shoe's upper is soft and pliable—leather, if possible. This rule may be ignored only when rigidity is important, as, for example, in the safety shoe.
- Choose a shoe that has a broad and fairly low heel. (This does not apply to high-fashion dress shoes such as the high-heeled pump.)
- Judge the rigidity or flexibility of the shank by bending the shoe. It should bend at the sole and not at the shank. Select a shoe shank that is appropriate to your specific needs. For instance, for mountain climbing the shoe's shank should be rigid, and for tennis it should be flexible.
- Make sure that the new shoe fits snugly at the heel and instep and that there is sufficient room at the front for extension of your toes.
- Any woman who wears high-heeled shoes should buy three pairs of shoes with different heel heights—flat, medium, and high—and rotate wearing them in succession. The variety of heel heights alternately stretch and relax the foot and leg muscles. The muscles of her calf would then stay limber, and her feet would be comfortable in both high heels and flats.
- Once you find shoes that fit just right, stay with that brand and with that width—perhaps even with that salesperson, if you have confidence in his or her ability to fit your feet with the proper footwear.

FOOT FACT

The average foot gets about two sizes longer when its owner stands up.

In addition, you should recognize that sneaker-style shoes are excellent as daily footgear. Almost all have advantageous features, and we recommend their use. The more expensive ones are likely to be less abusive to the feet.

The preceding rules can keep you from buying and wearing the wrong shoes. But no rules can cover all the special situations you might encounter. For in truth, every foot is unique. The left shoe of a pair might fit your left foot, but the right shoe might not fit your right foot comfortably, or vice versa. Make sure that both shoes fit you perfectly.

If you have a high instep, a short, plump foot, or a wide, short-toed foot, you might need to have shoes made especially for your feet. Why? Because the standardized lasts (foot-shaped wooden blocks over which new shoes are formed) used by shoe manufacturers for the mass market might not accommodate your foot shape. Combination lasts, which feature narrow heels and wide foreparts, can help with some problems, such as hammertoes and bunions; but in many cases they

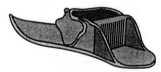

FIRST AMERICAN GALOSHES
1760-1780

Footnotes on the History of Sneakers

- The word "sneaker" was invented to describe the soundless shoes worn by sneak theives in England early in the twentieth century.
- The Prince of Wales (later to be King Edward VIII and then the Duke of Windsor) gave sneakers respectability when he toured the United States in 1920 and was seen wearing a pair of rubber footgear at a fashionable sporting event. They were the same sort of shoes worn by baseball players while stealing bases.
- The first crude sneakers were invented by the jungle natives of Brazil. A European expedition exploring the Amazon in 1736 found the Indians wearing shoes that had been made by dipping their feet into bowls of sap from a native tree and then standing in front of a fire until the sap hardened on their feet.
- The first "civilized" sneaker, made of sateen with elkskin trim and rubber soles, appeared in 1868. It was promptly adopted by the idle rich of Europe as a "croquet sandal," according to foot historian William Rossi. This civilized sneaker became the official "tennis shoe" in 1881 shortly after the game was invented in England.
- In the United States, Converse, then known as the Converse Rubber Shoe Company, produced its first sneaker—for lawn tennis—in 1908 and two years later was turning out 4,000 pairs a day.
- Sneakers were renamed athletic shoes in 1979, the year they broke the $50 price barrier. Five years later, some athletic shoes reached the $100 mark.
- Basketball shoes, which came along in 1910, sold for $1.25 a pair in 1917.

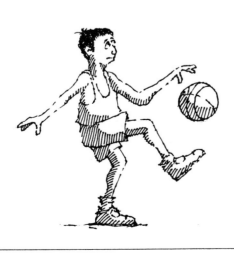 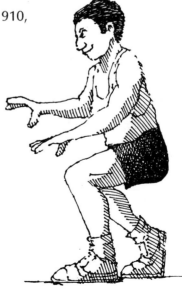

offer no solutions.

It's too bad that many persons who have difficulty in finding shoes that fit their feet properly assume that no help or relief is available; they continue to buy shoes that are made on standard lasts and continue to fall victim to injuries and chronic conditions that better-fitting shoes might have helped them avoid. They are unaware—because there is no one to advise them or because they do not ask—that there might be solutions.

Ultimately, the final decision rests with you. You can risk crippling yourself, or you can enjoy good foot health by following the simple rules for buying shoes. If, despite those rules, you still cannot get the correct footwear for your needs, then you had better consult a doctor of podiatric medicine.

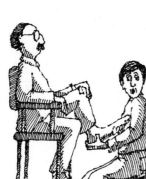

SIZING UP YOUR FEET

Shoes are measured by length and girth. The length is indicated numerically; the girth, or last, is indicated by letters. If you wear a size 7A, the seven indicates the length, the A the girth. Shoes for children range in size from 1 to 13, whereupon a new series of sizes begins for adults, again with size 1. Sizes in the United States are taken from the English measure. English shoe sizes were adopted by American manufacturers at the 1918 meeting of the National Boot and Shoe Manufacturers' Association.

The English standards measure whole sizes by thirds of an inch, beginning with $4\frac{1}{3}$. Thus, if a child's foot is $4\frac{1}{3}$ inches long, he will wear a size 1 shoe; if $4\frac{2}{3}$ inches long, a size 2, etc. The adult male sizes begin at $8\frac{2}{3}$ inches, for size 1, and proceed upward by thirds of an inch to size 13 for a foot that is $12\frac{2}{3}$ inches long.

Those measurements are also standard for the American shoe industry. However, they are not uniformly observed by every manufacturer. Thus, you can expect your shoe size to vary within a narrow range if you buy several different brands of footgear.

The breadth, or girth, of a shoe is known as the last. The standard last is C. Lasts vary from AAAAA (very narrow) to EEE (very broad); in exceptional cases, even wider or narrower lasts are used. The standard of difference between each last is one quarter of an inch. Lasts, like sizes, vary somewhat from manufacturer to manufacturer.

Even having a knowledge of shoe sizes and shoe materials won't ensure that your shoes will fit or will be correct for your feet. Shoes could have fit you just right when you bought them but be woefully inadequate by the time they are worn out; indeed, you might actually be damaging your feet by wearing that same pair of once well-fitting

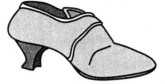

**WEDDING SLIPPER
ABOUT 1770**

shoes.

A little thought about the use to which you will put the footwear can also save your feet from harm. You should not buy shoes thoughtlessly. Examine them and make sure they are right for you before you have them wrapped to take home. Get them fitted correctly with the right sizing.

THE SHOE SALESPERSON'S ROLE

In addition to choosing the proper shoes for a particular task and fitting the feet individually, there is another problem: Is your shoe salesperson qualified to fit you?

In some cases, no.

Although it is understandable that a customer may know little about the function and requirements of the feet and what a pair of shoes can be expected to do, it is inexcusable when a shoe clerk is poorly informed.

Shoes can cause deformities. The clerk should therefore know enough to warn a customer when shoes are ill-suited or dangerous. A shoe clerk should not permit a customer to buy shoes that can be only harmful to him or her. Naturally, the clerk cannot forbid a customer from buying and wearing shoes that don't fit, but he or she can guide that purchaser to acquiring correct footgear—if the shoe salesperson knows what is right. Then, if the customer insists on buying inappropriate footgear, the salesperson can at least know that he or she did all that could be expected of a conscientious shoe clerk.

To do that much, however, the shoe clerk must be well informed on the products he or she sells. Rarely is that the case in today's marketplace.

We recommend that state legislatures remedy the situation by providing for the licensing of all shoe salespersons. If standards were set and if licensing examinations were given by state boards of health, the public would be assured that each shoe clerk was fully qualified. The clerk would know about shoe construction, shoe lasts and sizes, foot anatomy, foot measurement, and what constitutes a good fit. If such licensing was required, each salesperson who dispenses footgear would have to be trained minimally in those matters before he or she could secure a license to fit the shoes, upon which basic foot health depends.

Closely examined, our proposal is not extreme. With some other parts of the anatomy that require product or service—eyes and eyeglasses, for example—the fitter and the seller are each licensed by governmental authority. Minimum standards of knowledge and skill are set and enforced. Standards are maintained for hair service through

FOOT FACT

Shoe sizes were devised in England by King Edward II, who declared in 1324 that the diameter of one barleycorn—a third of an inch—would represent one full shoe size. Today, that's still true.

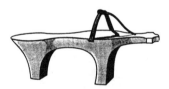

SANDAL OF SUMATRA 1800

the licensing of barbers and beauticians. If licensing can be done for those services, why not for the sellers of shoes, whose actions can influence the foot health of the public for months, perhaps years, to come?

A minimum licensing program would do much to prevent many of the foot problems and ailments that now afflict a vast amount of people. More than any other article of clothing, footwear potentially can cause considerable harm to the wearer. Any actions that could protect the public from such harm should be taken.

HIGH-HEELED, POINTED-TOE CULPRITS

Women suffer more often from foot problems than do men (or at least they see podiatrists more often than men do), and the reason they experience more discomfort can be traced directly to the shoes they wear. The crime of crippling women's feet is committed in shoe shops around the world; a major culprit is the shape of the shoes.

Most women's foot problems today are contributed to by two kinds of footgear: the high-heeled shoe and the pointed-toe shoe. Of course, high-heeled shoes have been worn for decades. Recently, the heels seem to have become higher than ever, and one result has been more cases of discomfort and deformed feet.

Common sense should tell us that nature never intended us to stand or walk on three-inch spike heels. The human foot does not have three-inch tapered heel bones! Nor did nature intend us to jam our toes into pointed-toe shoes. Our feet were created with rounded outlines. If you doubt what those types of shoes do to women's feet, then look at the feet that tread any public beach. Seldom can wearers of those shoes boast of lovely feet.

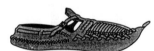

**APACHE INDIAN MOCCASIN
ABOUT 1870**

High-heeled shoes are not the only offenders. Even shoes for casual wear have been made with pointed toes. And men's styles, too, have been affected. As a result, podiatrists are seeing more ingrown toenails, corns, and bunions than ever—on boys and girls as well as on adults.

The square-toe, or bulldog, shoe is a variation of the pointed-toe style but is not much better. This style is deceptive. The pointed toe has been squared by lopping off the part of the shoe into which the toes cannot possibly fit. Although the shoes are tapered as sharply as before, the square end gives them an appearance of broadness. The purchaser thinks the shoe is more nearly shaped like the foot, but it is not.

The spike-heel, pointed-toe pump is one of the worst torture devices ever invented for the foot of man (make that woman). But its popularity continues, although nearly every woman will testify that it inflicts pain when she wears it.

Shoes with high heels, especially those higher than two inches, are to be condemned absolutely. Is that a severe judgment? You need only to try and stand an inexpensive, three-inch, narrow-diameter, spike-heel shoe upright on any flat surface. The shoe will wobble and fall at the slightest touch. There is no reason to believe the shoe will be more stable when you stand inside it. Put the shoe on, and try to balance yourself on that one foot. You will find it extremely difficult to do.

What actually happens to a woman's foot when she wears high-heeled, pointed-toe shoes? X-ray photographs of feet in pointed-toe pumps have been compared with photographs of the same feet bare. The comparison reveals that the high-heeled, pointed-toe pump compresses the toes by one-half to one inch. At the same time, the weight of the body causes the foot to slide forward and down into the shoe. The effect is distortion, contraction, overlapping, and compression of the entire foot structure, eventually causing toenail problems, bunions, corns, tired feet, and many other afflictions.

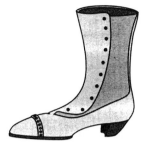

U.S. WOMAN'S SHOE 1900

PROBLEMS CAUSED BY EXTREME SHOE FASHIONS

The tapered-toe shoe tends to put undue pressure on the first, second, and fifth toes, along the fleshy folds of tissue at the sides of the nails. Such excessive pressure causes the edge of the nail to penetrate the flesh that is being pushed against it by the shoe, for the nail is often sharp as a knife. Consequently, although there might be no particular nail problem to start with, the pressure produces symptoms of inflammation. The inflammation can develop into callused nail grooves, a corn under the nail, or even an infection. The pain is the same as that from a true ingrown toenail.

Podiatrists find that capsulitis of the big toe joint is another acute problem. Capsulitis occurs when the capsule (the tissue surrounding the joint of the big toe) becomes stretched and distended by the forward motion of the foot as it comes downward in a three-inch spike heel. Excessive pressure on the first metatarsal joint strains the capsule, and the continued strain causes an acute inflammation with an influx of fluid and swelling.

The tapered-toe shoe also crowds the sesamoid bones (the two little seed-shaped bones beneath the first metatarsal), and that can lead to a condition known as dancer's foot. As the foot springs off when it takes a step, its sesamoid bones are squeezed by the narrowness of the tapered-toe shoe. They are pressed to one side, and as the foot strikes the ground, the sesamoid bones catch the weight at the wrong angle. Although the foot can take this a few times, the constant jarring effect from a long walk will produce an acute pain that is difficult to relieve, a pain that lingers even after the shoes have been removed.

A different problem—a bunion—develops when the sac of fluid in the bursa normally present at the big toe joint is squeezed and inflamed by an ill-fitting shoe. When the shoe squeezes the bursa, the first metatarsal tends to rotate on its long axis. As a result, the joint of the big toe rubs constantly against the upper leather of the woman's dress shoe. Continued pressure and friction cause redness, heat, swelling, and pain in the joint. That can happen in tapered-toe or square-toe shoes.

HOW TO PREVENT FOOT PRESSURES FROM DRESS SHOES

Some of the synthetic materials used for insoles in the newer shoe styles do not give enough cushioning to the feet. A leather insole is much better and, indeed, is recommended by us. It can be installed as a replacement insole to give your feet some relief. But, given the price of shoes and of separate insoles, you might be better off buying a shoe with a leather insole in the first place.

You can also secure relief by placing a thin platform beneath the lining of the shoe where the first metatarsal presses into the insole. The inserted pad will prevent the metatarsal from rotating. It will also act as a lever that holds the bone in position and keeps the foot balanced. The platform can be a piece of felt or cork or even quarter-inch-thick cardboard. To lift the lining, put in the pad, and paste the lining back is a simple procedure.

If all women who wear tapered-toe shoes were to take that simple action, then some of the symptoms podiatrists now see in their patients might never develop. Of course, the best solution is not to wear the tapered-toe shoe at all. A change in current fashion styles to a more sensible shoe would accomplish the same result.

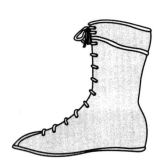

WOMAN'S BATHING SHOE
U.S.A. 1900

Some women do not have trouble with pointed-toe shoes—but only because their feet are naturally tapered. Women who have long toes say this shoe style is heavenly for them, but few women are so fortunate.

OVERCOMING THE CRIPPLING EFFECTS OF FASHIONS

It probably is obvious by now that the shoes we buy and wear can have important effects upon our health—not only the health of our lower limbs but of our bodies overall. If we choose our shoes wisely, we can reduce the number of problems we have with our feet and the rest of our skeleton. But if we accept and wear just any shoes, then we can multiply the problems, especially those caused primarily by what the designers designate as being in vogue.

Not everyone follows the fashions so readily accepted by the masses. Some, such as the wealthy superfashionites who can afford to live above the crowd, create their own fashions. Others cannot afford to buy every new style. In between those two groups are the vast majority, trapped and unprotesting, who purchases any shoe the fashionable shoe designer offers.

Still, even fashion has two faces. One is ornamental, frivolous, and decorative. The other is functional, physiological, and adaptive. The truly creative shoe designer should combine the two into a product that the public can wear safely and fashionably. The shoe designers who set the fashions should consult their own foot doctors to find out how flexible and mobile the feet are and how far one can, or should, go in the design of new fashions.

In this age of new materials and new creative opportunities, shoe designs need not be limited to the old malfunctional patterns. If a shoe designer wants to be truly creative, he or she should accept these challenges:

- Design a shoe with a removable insole. The foot covering would become a bit larger when the insole is removed and smaller when it is restored, helping feet that have become swollen, for many feet do swell after considerable walking on paved streets.
- Design a shoe for each of the various foot types—high-instep foot, short-toed foot, and the like—especially for the three types of trouble-prone feet described on page fourteen. Each shoe could be fitted by matching a tracing of the customer's foot to a presized pattern.
- Design a shoe with a moldable insole that would take on the form of the foot. The insole would be soft and pliable and would change shape along with the foot as each step is taken.
- Design a shoe made entirely of straps so that each dimension could be varied to fit different feet.

The challenge is to the designer. Comfortable, beautiful, and safe shoe styles are possible. Shoes can be artistic without crippling the feet. To the designer who creates shoes that will be a boon rather than a curse to the wearer, mankind will not merely be grateful but will surely bring him or her great rewards.

FOOT FACT

Some running shoes have replaceable soles, so the bottoms can be quickly stripped off and changed to suit the terrain.

4. *Pain and Surgery*

EVEN a faithfully followed, sensible, foot care program won't always prevent every foot trouble. Problems might still develop, and pain could persist despite the diligent application of self-help remedies.

WHEN THE PAIN PERSISTS

It is usually pain that brings a victim of foot maladies to seek to correct the problem. Various ailments such as recurring corns, tailor's bunions (prominences over the fifth metatarsal joints), bony spurs under the heels, and some other foot troubles rarely go away by themselves. You have to help yourself or seek treatment by a doctor. Therapeutic efforts by a doctor of podiatric medicine skilled in surgical, mechanical, or other corrective techniques are intended to rid the patient of pain, of course, but more importantly, they aim to find the basic cause of the discomfort and correct it.

One of the mysteries of pain is its contrariness. There is no way to tell how serious a health problem is simply by the severity of the pain. The pain of glaucoma is quiescent, so much so that it gives no hint that the sufferer is in danger of becoming blind. The inflammatory pain of an ingrown toenail is so insistent that it makes it difficult to concentrate on anything else, but it certainly isn't life-threatening. The inflammatory pain of a ruptured appendix is about equal in intensity to that of the ingrown toenail, but the appendicitis causing that pain can kill. The ingrown toenail only cripples.

Pain is clearly no simple or single sensation. The term is merely a label describing one's discomfort; it is a convenient way to define feelings, symptoms, reactions, and forms of personal hurt. To the average person, pain is the symptom and the disease. But to the foot doctor, the pain experienced by his patient is not the disease; rather, it is the symptom of an abnormality in some part of the foot.

The presence of pain has severe psychological overtones, too. To avoid surgical pain, hospitalization, long recuperative time, high financial costs, and excessive disability, some people will take self-help measures to get rid of their malady. Alternatively, others will travel long distances to be treated by a doctor who gives them permanent relief.

In some cases, alleviation of the pain or correction of the underlying foot problem will require surgery. Standard surgical procedures can help, but there is another option.

AMBULATORY PODIATRIC SURGERY

The results of podiatric surgery performed with techniques borrowed from orthopedic surgery are not always satisfactory. Some podiatrists who belong to the American College of Foot Surgeons use dramatically long incisions, which allow them to get their instruments into the tissues, sinews, joints, and other structures of the foot. But such incisions bring their own set of complications. Big surgical openings require closure with lots of threaded stitches. The more sutures needed to close a surgical wound, the greater the possibility of infection.

A less painful form of foot surgery, as well as a method that required a shorter recuperation period, had been needed for a long time. The right set of skilled procedures, but less costly in terms of hospital care, was crying to be found. We are lucky to have it now.

In recent years, Americans annually have paid $500 billion for health care. And the costs each year continue to escalate. Can we lower health care costs yet not stint the patients in getting the finest available services from our health professionals? Yes, we can. Doctors who practice ambulatory foot surgery have contributed one of the ways.

Ambulatory foot surgeons have developed minimal-incision techniques that are just as good as or better than the older methods. The correction of foot deformities once required large openings, long cuts, a spreading of the tissue layers, sometimes metal pins and plaster casts, and many sutures for closure of the wound; but ambulatory foot surgeons have perfected less-traumatic procedures.

Ambulatory podiatric surgery makes only tiny openings in the skin of a foot that needs correction. The involved region is not entirely exposed. Instead, specially constructed tools similar to those adapted for microsurgery are inserted into the tiny surgical openings so that only the immediate problem area is involved. Abnormal bone growths, unsightly toenails, benign tumors, cysts, crooked toes, heel spurs, and other foot troubles are corrected in a manner virtually pain-free.

Ambulatory foot surgery, a subbranch of minimal-incision surgery, results in much less discomfort than the old-fashioned surgical methods produce. Now, patients are able to leave the doctor's office (the surgery is not available in hospitals) under their own power. Ambulatory foot surgery is so atraumatic and usually so painless, particularly if mild painkillers are taken, that no bed confinement is required. Often, the foot patient can return to work right from the surgical chair.

There is precedent in medicine for achieving maximum benefit through the most minimal of incisions. Cataracts are corrected that way. Facial features are altered through plastic surgical techniques using the tiniest cuts. Cryosurgery of the brain to correct Parkinson's disease is done through the smallest of skull openings. Aids no bigger than a pin are microsurgically implanted to restore hearing to the deaf and sight to the blind. So it is with minimal incisions in ambulatory foot surgery. The ability to walk in comfort is being restored to the lame, the crippled, and the deformed.

CUTTING DOWN ON HOSPITAL COSTS

Office-based minimal-incision surgery definitely cuts costs and precludes patients from unnecessarily taking up hospital beds for the seriously ill. Since ambulatory foot surgery is an office procedure, it requires fewer health personnel such as nurses, cooks, dietitians, orderlies, maintenance people, and so many others. The sheer reduction in personnel lowers the operation's cost not only to the patient, but also to his or her health insurance carrier and to society.

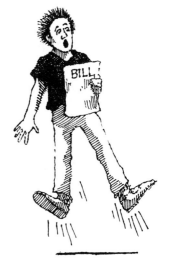

Abram Plon, doctor of podiatric medicine and former president of the Academy of Ambulatory Foot Surgeons, has said, "The greatest cost factor in medical or surgical care is the hospital bill. In the majority of cases of foot surgery, hospitalization is unnecessary. An estimated $100 million annually could be saved if operations were done in the podiatrist's office instead of in a hospital. Based on national hospital cost figures, a foot surgery patient could save as much as $500 a day by having his operation performed in the doctor's office.

"For psychological reasons, the patient not only does better at home after a foot operation, but the operative wound usually heals faster."

A medical procedure is considered surgery as long as an instrument is inserted under the skin. The size or length of the incision is not a

Treating Systemic Disorders Through Foot Acupuncture

"That a needle stuck into one's foot should improve the functioning of one's liver is obviously incredible. The only trouble is that, as a matter of empirical fact, it does happen." So wrote novelist Aldous Huxley in 1962, in his foreword to Dr. Felix Mann's *Acupuncture: Cure of Many Diseases.*

For thousands of years, the Chinese have used the power of the foot for more than walking. They have created a system of health care called acupuncture, which uses key points on the foot and elsewhere to treat disorders affecting other parts of the body. For instance, swelling might appear on the inside or outside of a painful but uninjured ankle. The outer ankle is connected to the bladder meridian; the inner ankle belongs to the kidney meridian. Acupuncturists know that inner ankle swelling indicates kidney malfunction. Their treatment involves using electrical stimulation or moxabustion to heat certain ankle points (Tai ch'i #3, Ta Chung #4, and Shui Ch'uan #5), a spleen meridian point (San Yin Chiao #6), and specific conception meridian points (Shang Kuan #13 and Kuan Yuan #4).

Patients receiving acupuncture treatments for the bladder or kidney problems indicated by swollen ankles will also be advised to eliminate from their diets all coffee, juice, cold foods, and cold liquids. The acupuncture community considers only two teas safe to drink when the kidneys are impaired: ginseng and oolong. Acupuncture is administered twice weekly for about six treatments. Soaking in warm water before retiring at night assists in the improvement.

Doctor of podiatric medicine G. Wayne Jower wrote in the February 1983 issue of the *Journal of Current Podiatric Medicine* that acupuncture points on foot deformities correlate with disorders in the rest of the body. Dr. Jower's article clearly designates the exact acupuncture points and the foot anatomy at which they are located. For instance, one can overcome gastric spasm and acute gastroenteritis by stimulating acupoint #8 in the arch; or one can eliminate dysentery and diarrhea with action on acupoints #5 and #6 in the same general foot area.

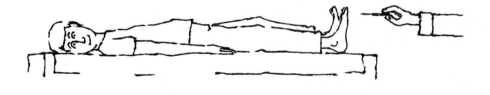

determining factor. Health insurance companies recognize this and compensate for ambulatory operations as long as they eliminate the offending problem.

Health insurance carriers love to see patients avoid hospitalization, thereby saving the insurance company much money. Ambulatory surgery, using minimal-incision techniques to remove a corn or any other foot lesion, requires no hospitalization. It is an in-office procedure done by the podiatrist.

Hospitals are expensive; still, some people enter them even for corn removals. Such an elective procedure points up the advantages of in-office surgery. If done in the hospital, it involves admission and the associated entry charge. Next come expensive tests, including an unnecessary chest X-ray and an extraneous electrocardiogram, to protect the hospital from liability. A complete patient history and physical examination are required even if they have been performed recently by the family doctor.

FOOT FACT

The left foot is usually slightly larger than the right in right-handed people, and vice versa in lefties.

The patient has to enter the hospital a day in advance for those tests, so a room charge is added. Piled on is the charge for use of the operating room and instruments. There is another charge for use of the recovery room while the anesthetic wears off. Charges for two more days are tacked on for the patient's recuperation in his hospital room. Casts, splints, bandages, and medicines are all added to the total bill. The surgeon slips in his fee; the anesthesiologist adds his. Indeed, even if the surgeon administers a local anesthetic, the anesthesiologist must stand by with an intravenous blood line ready, just in case of an emergency. If any other health professional checks the patient, there will be a charge for the visit.

Walter J. McNerney, former president of the Blue Cross and Blue Shield associations, has expressed outrage and shock that those costs and others less obvious can easily add up to $3,500, even for a minor foot operation. Blue Cross/Blue Shield aggressively encourages walk-in and walk-out ambulatory surgery as a cost-saving mechanism.

HOLISTIC APPROACH

The term "holistic" describes ambulatory foot surgery's minimal-incision method. The procedure not only corrects the patient's physical disability, but its gentleness relieves fear and tension. Ambulatory foot surgery lifts the spirit by freeing the individual from deformity and pain. Although the terms "surgery" and "holistic" are by nature contradictory, the newest methods of foot care turn holistic foot surgery into reality.

With ambulatory foot surgery, the time that the patient must wait to undergo the operation is considerably reduced. He recuperates

amid familiar surroundings and eats familiar foods and not the gar-
bage-type materials served up by dietitians practicing on patients in
hospitals. Collectively, the individual benefits of having a foot correction done out of the hospital constitute a favorable psychological
picture. It is a true holistic approach to taking care of the entire person
while focusing on the disability in a foot.

Part Two

Conspicuous
Foot Problems:
Causes and Treatments

5. *Toenail Troubles*

THE toenails, those hard, shiny, translucent plates at the ends of your toes, are designed by nature to protect the delicate structures residing within your toe tips. Under normal conditions they do the job of protecting, for their strength and rigidity shield nerves, tiny blood vessels, and toe bones. But the toenails, especially on the big toes, can become a source of discomfort and even dangerous infection.

SOURCES OF TOENAIL TROUBLES

On a natural terrain, a person who walks barefoot exposes his toes to many hazards that might greatly harm his feet if they had no toenails. When he wears shoes, however, the toes and toenails are protected against most traumas. It would seem logical to assume that little harm could be done to the toenails and that they could scarcely be the source of foot troubles if shoes are worn. Not so! Even in shoes, and often because of shoes, the toenails get damaged.

The most obvious source of toenail injury is the impact from a falling object. Where an obviously hazardous situation exists, it is common sense to take precautions. It is not unusual in certain industries for employers to require their workers to wear steel-capped safety shoes or boots; many employers even provide them. But in everyday situations, protecting the feet, and in particular the toes, from falling objects requires vigilance.

FOOT FACT

Toenails grow only a third to half as fast as fingernails. After a toenail is removed, it might take six to eight months for the new toenail to grow in completely.

45

The familiar causes of toenail problems are short shoes and short stockings—shoes and stockings not long enough to fit properly along the length of the foot. Excessive perspiration, improper nail cutting, and fungus infections also can cause toenail problems. To those causes must be added congenital malformations, adverse familial traits, systemic diseases (such as diabetes and arthritis), and tissue stress (in the overweight individual).

The most frequently encountered toenail troubles are ingrown nails, club nails, fungus infections, and callused nail grooves. Primarily they are brought on by the shoes you wear or the way you care, or neglect to care, for your feet. Pain or severe discomfort accompanies those problems. However, they can be treated, either by you at home using methods that come easily to hand or by a podiatrist who is skilled in foot surgery.

INGROWN TOENAIL

Of all toenail afflictions, the ingrown nail is the most common and painful. It occurs when one or both of the lateral edges of the nail penetrates the skin and cuts into the soft flesh of the toe. Unless quickly corrected, an ingrown nail can result in severe complications, progressing to simple inflammation, serious infection, ulceration, gangrene, and even death. Ingrown toenails are frequently at the inflammation or infection stage when treated by podiatrists. That is chiefly because anyone who suffers from it is seldom able to endure the pain and usually seeks aid before a more serious complication develops.

Although an ingrown nail can affect anyone, it occurs most often in persons between the ages of ten and thirty. Teenagers seem especially susceptible, perhaps because they do more walking than grown-ups or because they disregard the early warnings that adults will heed.

Any toe might suffer from an ingrown nail, but the big toe, because of its prominence and length, is involved most often. The agents responsible are improper cutting of the nails, hereditary effects, and tight shoes and stockings. Short footwear can exert pressure upon the big toe, press directly on the toenail grooves, and force the outside edge of the nail into the flabby nail fold.

In small children, an ingrown toenail might be traced—strange as it might seem—to tight clothing, leotards, sleepers, or other bedclothes. The subtle but prolonged pressure that those articles of clothing exert on the toenails as the child thrusts his feet forward can lead to serious problems in adulthood.

If a person has an inherited tendency toward nails with extreme curvature, the soft tissue of the fleshy folds might grow over the nail plate—and then the nail would grow inward. An overweight person

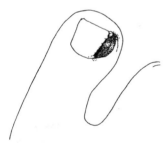

Figure 5.1
A toenail grows inward into the fleshy folds of this big toe. Fluid is starting to extrude from the acutely inflamed area. There is redness, swelling, a feeling of heat, and continuous pain, especially when the toe is touched.

who has chubby toes might also suffer from an ingrown nail that results from the fleshy folds' covering the nail plate.

The most frequent cause of ingrown nails, however, is injudicious cutting of the toenail using scissors or, worse, tearing off the nail corner with one's fingers. A few days after such self-administered "bathroom surgery," inflammation can appear at the offended corner of the nail. At first, there is some discoloration, a mild swelling, and the escape of a little fluid. (See Figure 5.1.)

If those signs are disregarded, infection sets in. Pus forms, and redness increases. Then, as the toe balloons, the pain starts. Sometimes, a bloody mass of material known as proud flesh appears at the lateral edge of the toenail between the nail plate and the nail groove. (See Figure 5.2.) Proud flesh is acutely painful and, when irritated or injured, bleeds readily.

At that point, most sufferers seek medical aid. If the ingrown nail goes untreated, a dangerous infection can spread along the whole toe, and red streaks could appear along the top of the foot. If treatment is not given at that time, the infection can enter the blood stream and proceed farther up the leg. A general physical weakness, accompanied by chills, fever, nausea, vomiting, and diarrhea, is liable to set in. Even gangrene might begin, and the battle the doctor must then fight is to save as much of the toe, foot, or leg as possible. Fortunately, few people allow the complications to go that far.

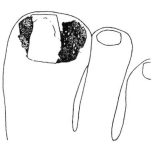

Figure 5.2
Proud flesh has formed in the outside lateral corner of this red-hot big toe. The nail also has proud flesh beginning to form on the inside lateral corner. The corners have been cut at an angle, but the toenail growing out from the matrix is still cutting into the fleshy folds, causing acute inflammation and pain.

REMEDIES FOR INGROWN TOENAIL

Treatment of the ingrown toenail by a podiatric surgeon involves removing the offending portion of the toenail, reducing the inflammation, and controlling the infection. In severe cases, a foot doctor might administer or prescribe antibiotics.

Various surgical procedures sometimes are used to eliminate chronic ingrown toenails. The podiatrist removes a portion of the nail, a portion of the underlying nail bed, some of the adjacent soft tissues, and even a part of the growth center. Minimal-incision surgery is effective for permanently eliminating the corners of the matrix so that nail edges growing inward do not cut into fleshy toe folds as the toenail grows forward. Electrical cauterization, chemical cauterization, or surgical excision help the health professional remove the corners of the patient's nail growth center forever.

You can help yourself at home if you are experiencing the very beginning of a toenail's digging laterally into the toe's soft tissues. Take some drugstore collodion liquid, and coat a wisp of cotton with it. Then slip the resulting moistened material into the space between the nail and the fleshy fold. As the collodion dries, the cotton firms and acts as

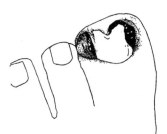

Figure 5.3
Making a V-cut does not
prevent ingrown toenail, as
depicted in the above art.

a wedge between the toenail and the fleshy fold. So, as the sharp edge of the nail grows, it will move past the toe's protruding flesh and thus avoid cutting into the soft parts.

According to an old wives' tale, cutting a V in the middle of a toenail will prevent it from growing inward. In truth, a V-cut is of little value since the nail grows from the matrix, not from the front, and the V-cut does not cause the sides of the nail to grow toward the middle. An ingrown toenail is likely to develop, along with proud flesh and infection, despite the V-cut. (See Figure 5.3.)

To avoid the problem of ingrown toenails, file the nail margins thin with an emery board to reduce the pressure on them, trim the nails straight across with toenail clippers, and clean the grooves with an orangewood stick. If despite following such precautions you suffer from an ingrown toenail, see a podiatrist at once for appropriate professional treatment.

CLUB NAIL

Persons over sixty years of age sometimes have thick, ugly, deformed toenails, a condition that can be symptomatic of a systemic disease, such as tuberculosis or syphilis. The nails of the hands and feet can indicate the state of one's health. Psoriasis, circulatory conditions, lung involvements, or coronary disease might be suspected when toenails are shiny, flecked, crumbly, or raised.

More frequently, injury alone causes the toenails to become discolored, elongated, or thickened. Those conditions might appear after the toes have received a blow from a falling object or have been stubbed on a piece of furniture.

Overgrown toenails are known as club nails. They can become extremely hard and curl under the toes to give the shape of a ram's horn. (See Figure 5.4.)

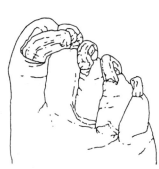

Figure 5.4
Ram's horn toenails have
developed on all the toes
of this right foot. Club nails
of this nature develop out
of foot neglect. Older folk
especially are predisposed
to club nails, because
frequently they lack the
strength to cut through their
hard and horny toenails.

Reduction of club nails does not have to be painful. You can do it yourself with a nail file, or you might use a revolving drill that holds a small sandpaper disk. The drill is similar to a tool used for detailed woodworking. Podiatrists routinely use such an instrument in practice, as do dentists. But before using the file or drill, first lubricate and soften the nail by rubbing it with warm mineral oil or olive oil and then use a strong nail clippers to cut as much of it as you comfortably can without hurting yourself.

Podiatrists usually smooth club nails and give them a more pleasing appearance. However, the main purpose in reducing overgrown nails is to remove pressure from the nail grooves and thereby eliminate the source of discomfort. Reduction also leaves more space for toe movement in the shoe. More room in the shoe will likely relieve pressure and so prevent corns from forming on adjacent toes. A shoe salesperson who serves someone who suffers from club nails should advise the customer to wear shoes and hosiery that are long enough to allow free movement of the toes.

Minimal-incision surgery corrects club nail by removing the matrix, or growth center. The operation is performed in the podiatrist's office. Hospitalization is unnecessary. Using local anesthesia similar to what a dentist uses to numb your teeth and gums when filling a cavity, the foot doctor blocks sensation into the end of the toe. That way, your nail can be removed to allow access to the toenail's growth center.

The surgeon puts a cauterizing solution in the space under the fleshy overhang that had held down the now-removed toenail. Cauterization eliminates the matrix so that no nail will grow on that toe anymore. When the dressing comes off the end of the toe in about a week, the flesh covering the toe end hardens and firms. It looks just like a toenail is present, but none is there. Some women even apply nail polish to the toe top, though no nail is present.

FUNGUS INFECTION

Research by a pharmaceutical company indicates that one out of every four persons over the age of thirty who visit podiatrists has a toenail infection caused by a fungus.

Fungus toenail is caused by parasitic fungi, yeasts, or molds, all of which grow as ringworm on the toenails. Fungi are prevalent in shoes, which, because they are the only item of clothing never thoroughly cleaned on the inside, are a constant source of infection and reinfection.

A nail with a fungus infection appears dry, lusterless, scaly, and streaked; it is raised from the nail bed and has a gray-yellow-brown, worm-eaten look. Part or all of the nail can be affected. As the infection progresses, it works back toward the nail root, causing destruction of the nail as it travels. A bumpiness and moth-eaten appearance will likely result, and only one nail on the foot need be involved. (See Figure 5.5.)

Because a fungus infection of the toenails is painless, the average person usually but erroneously pays no attention to the crumpled appearance of his toenails. To ignore the condition, though, might be to compound the danger, for the infected toenails would become an ever present site from which the more severe symptoms of athlete's foot could develop. There is also a danger that the fingernails might become infected if the sufferer scratches or soothes his toes with his fingers.

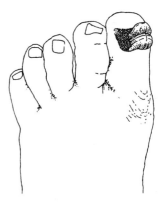

Figure 5.5
The big toenail on this left foot has been invaded by the fungus infection *Candida albicans*, a common yeast organism that produces nail distortion and the nail's moth-eaten appearance.

COMBATTING FUNGUS TOENAIL

In treating a fungus infection, podiatrists remove the crusted, powdery substance that forms around the thickened nail and file the nail thin. They might ionize the area with copper sulphate (a curative treatment that has been used with some success). Fungicides are applied directly onto and under the infected nail. Griseofulvin, a drug taken internally, might be prescribed to kill the fungus.

In some cases, the nails become so infected that they have to be removed entirely. When that happens, treatment must be directed to the nail bed and to the growth center from which the new nail will grow. The matrix is not destroyed, as it is with club nails, but instead is treated with anti-fungal remedies.

For self-help, we suggest that you go to the health food store and acquire an aged garlic extract called Kyolic, available in capsules, liquid, and tablets. Take it internally so that yeast overgrowth in your gut, the primary source of yeast infection on your toenails, is killed. You can also apply liquid aged garlic extract directly onto your invaded toenails.

CALLUSED NAIL GROOVE

Given the right circumstances, a corn or callus readily forms at the side of the toenail. It develops in the nail groove, where the free edge of the toenail meets the flesh. Such a callus, which often gets mistaken for an ingrown nail, is nature's way of protecting the fleshy part of the toe from continued friction against the nail plate. If a callus does not form to protect the nail fold when a tight shoe presses against it, then the nail usually will cut into the flesh and produce symptoms and signs characteristic of ingrown toenail.

How to treat a callused nail groove? If there is no discomfort, your corn or callus in the groove probably should be left alone. If pain does develop, you can help yourself by soaking the affected toe in hot soapy water or rubbing it with a cotton applicator and mineral oil, olive oil, or oil of vitamin E to soften the hard skin at the nail groove.

On the other hand, if enough thick callus has accumulated to cause deformity of the nail and inflammation of the toe, then the services of a podiatrist should be sought to bring the problem under control. (See Figure 5.6.)

Men's dress shoes, in particular the pointed-toe Italian styles, tend to cause calluses in the nail grooves. Women's pointed-toe shoes, of course, also bring on such calluses.

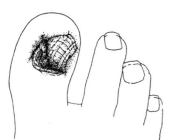

Figure 5.6
Callus formation in the nail groove of the big right toe has caused abnormal growth of the toenail. The callused nail groove appears similar to a fungus, and the big toenail has the start of a ram's horn look to it, but the toe's problem is merely callus. The callused nail groove is producing pressure pain in the toe.

PREVENTING TOENAIL DISCOMFORT AND DISTORTION

Observing two simple procedures will prevent many uncomfortable or distorted toenail conditions:

- Cut your toenails short, but keep them square by cutting straight across. Don't round the edges.
- Use professional-type toenail clippers. Avoid scissors for nail cutting, and never tear your toenails.

There is little in the human anatomy that does not serve a specific purpose. Just as the hair on the head has its function—to hold together the scalp—the toenails have theirs: to protect the bones and nerves of the toes. Yet, because we wear shoes, the toenails are a potential source of annoyance. However, we can protect ourselves from the problems they might cause by caring for our toenails properly.

6. *Corn Tortures*

WHILE hardening of the skin at points of friction can serve the purpose of protecting delicate structures in the flesh beneath, some kinds of skin hardening—such as corns—serve no purpose at all. They just hurt! But you can restore yourself to foot comfort even if you have one or more of the many types of corns.

Corns are probably the most common ailment to which the human foot is subject. About forty percent of all persons who visit foot doctors do so initially because of a corn problem. Fully half of the nation's women—and women make up eighty percent of podiatric patients—eventually will seek relief from the agonizing pain resulting from corns.

The scientific name designating a corn is *heloma.* It would seem that a large part of the adult population at some time or other suffers from heloma pain. Frequently heard from foot pain sufferers is, "My corns are killing me!" There is scarcely another word relating to the foot that will bring forth as much sympathy as the uttered word "corn." Nearly everyone has either had a heloma or knows somebody who has suffered ill effects from the malady. There are half a dozen types of corns, but only two can be considered common.

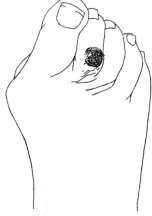

Figure 6.1
A hard corn on the top of the second toe shows the corn's central eye, along with the inflamed flesh surrounding it. The corn sticks upward and is swollen and painful.

HARD CORNS

The hard corn (heloma durum) is a growth of horny skin, generally located on the tops of the toes. It is easily distinguished from the normal tissue that surrounds it. There is a central radix, or eye, of hard gray skin, around which will be found a painful, raised, yellow, inflammatory ring of skin and flesh.

A hard corn can form on top of any of the five toes, but the second toe is most generally the site for the prominence. (See Figure 6.1.) The fifth toe often suffers from hard corn growth, too, and can cause the shoe-wearing victim agony with each step.

Hard corns are caused by friction and pressure, both of which in large measure are caused by the design of modern footgear. Hard corns develop on narrow surfaces of the skin, usually at a toe joint. The skin, although stocking clad, rubs repeatedly against the inside of the shoe, hardens, and dies. As the friction and pressure continue, extra skin grows continuously, layer after layer, leaving even less room between the shoe and the foot, and the developing corn is pressed more firmly against the underlying soft tissues and bone. The irritation and the pain increase as the hard corn grows outward.

The pain of a hard corn can also arise from bursitis, which is the inflammation of a bursa. The bursa is a sac of fluid beneath the skin; it ordinarily protects parts of the body against irritation from friction. The constant friction and pressure of shoe leather against skin and bone might produce beneath the hard corn an adventitious bursa that puts pressure on the sensory nerve endings. The pressure causes discomfort that varies from a dull, mild ache to a sharp, stabbing pain. Such pains increase if the corn is further irritated by tight shoes.

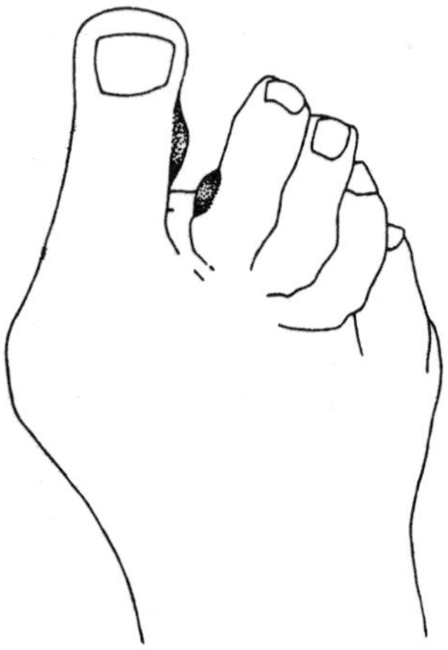

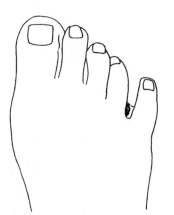

Figure 6.2
Soft corns can form where two toes rub together. Two such soft corns are shown on the adjoining inside areas of the first and second toes.

SOFT CORNS

The soft corn (heloma molle) most often occurs between the toes and is stimulated to grow by one toe's pinpoint pressure against another. The pain occurs because a bone prominence sticks upward from underneath the skin. Pressure from the bone within causes layers of skin to form over the prominence until it comes into proximity with its mate on the opposite toe, which also has a bone prominence. Their juxtaposition has them rubbing each other. It's likely that two soft corns will form, one on each toe, as a result of their friction rubs. (See Figure 6.2.)

The constant toe friction makes the adjoining pockets of skin die, grow thickened, become inflamed, and hurt with each step. You need not even wear shoes to feel the pain of soft corns, especially if they have developed between the toes. (See Figure 6.3.)

Figure 6.3
A soft corn developed between the fourth and fifth toes of this foot when two bones rubbed together within the flesh, pinching skin on the outside and deadening the skin tissue.

OTHER CORNS

Distal corns (heloma distallus), which develop at the tips of the toes, occur when toe contractures have the toes hammering downward to the ground with each step. (See Figure 6.4.)

Blood corns (heloma vasculare) have tiny blood vessels embedded in their centers. They form as a result of injury that extends into some of the underlying tissue.

Nerve corns (heloma nervosum) are round, hard, thick layers of skin in which overgrowths of nerve filaments extend very close to the surface. When any pressure is applied, the filaments cause excruciating pain.

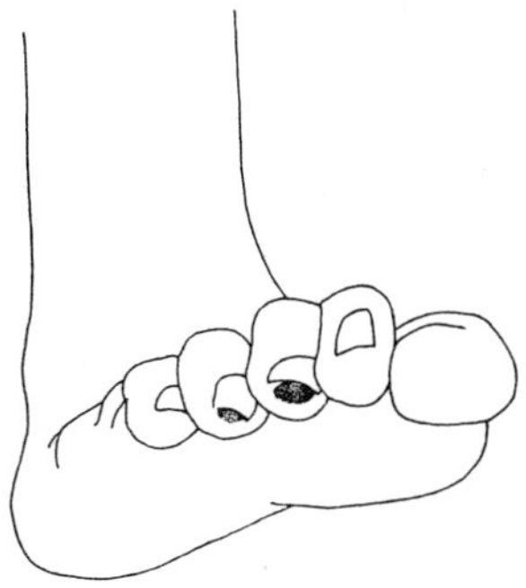

Seed corns (heloma milliare) are probably the least troublesome type. Pain might not even be present, depending on whether the corn is at a soft and pliable site (no pain) or over a prominence of bone (painful). Seed corns are the size of pinheads and usually appear on the bottom of the foot, especially around the heel, but they can occur on the toes, too. (See Figure 6.5.) But even when on the foot soles, where all the skin is thick, if a number of them form close together, they can become annoying, creating the same sensation as that of a pebble in your shoe. Seed corns are sometimes associated with the fungal growth of athlete's foot.

Arthritis can be an indirect cause of corns. It can deform the joints of the toes, leading to abnormally prominent joints that contact the inside of the shoe. The pressure and friction then produce a corn. Arthritic spurs can also form on, in, or around the toe joints and contribute to the deformity.

Persons who suffer from corns often complain that their extra skin outgrowths hurt much more when the weather changes. The complaints are justified. As a storm approaches, the air becomes filled with moisture and the atmospheric pressure goes down. The fluid in the inflamed bursa beneath a corn then attempts to rise from an area of high density beneath the skin to an area of lower density in the air. The bursal fluid expands, but because it cannot flow through the thick skin, the pressure on the surrounding nerves increases. The skin is stretched, and more pain is felt by the victim.

THREE WAYS TO DEFEAT CORNS

There are three ways to avoid suffering from painful corns: find temporary relief, receive a permanent cure, and prevent them in the first place.

Most important is prevention. Preventive treatment begins with recognizing that shoes pressing your toes together are the prime cause of corns. You cannot very well go without footwear, since you need protection for your feet. However, you can exercise wisdom in choosing shoes that fit your feet properly. Buy shoes that do not rub or pinch the toes. Before buying, walk in the shoes for a while to uncover flaws.

Figure 6.4
Distal corns, especially at the tip of the third toe, developed because of toe contracture and the subsequent hammering of toe tips on the sole of the shoe during walking.

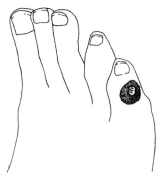

Figure 6.5
A seed corn on the top of this fifth toe can cause some distress.

Once you have found a shoe style that you can wear in absolute comfort, continue to wear that type of shoe. If you have confidence that a particular shoe salesperson fits you correctly, then continue to purchase your footgear from him or her.

The ideal footwear to avoid corns might be molded shoes. They are made from plaster replicas of your feet and are shaped to fit your feet exactly. When you wear them, the friction and pressure that can cause corns are completely eliminated.

If, like so many people, you do not find molded shoes acceptable—after all, they're shaped like feet, and most people's feet are ugly—then keep in mind that whatever kind of shoes you wear must fit properly to give you maximum comfort.

Corns can be relieved, cured, or prevented. If you choose to ignore foot comfort and insist on wearing fashionable footwear, then you can expect to suffer. Obviously, there are social events that demand conformity to modes of dress. At such times, you might feel it necessary to wear narrow, uncomfortable shoes. But do not wear them often—if you wish to avoid pain from corns. The choice is yours: sensible, practical shoes and freedom from pain; or uncomfortable, fashionable shoes and the presence of pain. As long as you choose fashion over comfort, expect to have corns, which must be treated either by yourself or, preferably, by a foot doctor.

If there is pressure or friction when walking, you might be able to correct it by altering the mechanics inside the shoe. You might get relief by taking any or all of these steps:

- Add a thin insole.
- Raise the heel with a 1/8-inch felt pad.
- Stretch the upper leather with a shoe-stretching device.
- Paste a strip of moleskin or podiatry felt around the heel seat.
- Push out the shoe's toe front just a little by slipping it over a broom handle and pressing downward.

Those are old tricks usually performed in a shoe store's back room to make a shoe fit better and clinch a sale when the correct size for a potential customer is absent from stock and can't readily be acquired.

TEMPORARY SELF-HELP CORN RELIEF

Temporary self-help does nothing to prevent the corns from growing in again later at the same place. However, it does provide you with immediate relief from discomfort.

Home treatment consists of shielding and padding the corn and the area of inflammation surrounding it. The principle behind padding a corn is to transfer the pressure of the shoe from a painful spot to one free from pain. Although padding corns is an art mastered by podiatrists in their professional training, any drugstore will sell you podiatry felt or moleskin—soft, pliable materials with adhesive on one side—to pad the corns. If you place a half-moon-shaped pad, one-eighth to one-quarter of an inch thick and sliced thin on its edges, just behind the corn, you will protect it against further irritation. To keep the pad from rolling up as it rubs against the stocking, attach it to the skin with adhesive tape. That is good treatment—except for persons who have diabetes or poor circulation. Then, the tape could damage the skin.

To relieve the pain of the inflammation beneath a hard corn, take a pad slightly thicker than the corn, make a cutout in the pad, and place a small dose of soothing medication in the center. (See Figure 6.6.) Emollient skin oil, such as what you use to keep hands soft and smooth, might suffice. Also, a non-prescription ointment for burns—one that contains no acid—is good at providing comfort from corns. Cover the medication with a wisp of cotton, and loosely wrap the pad with half-inch-wide strips of adhesive tape.

Beware of trying to treat your corns by cutting them. Cutting corns is hazardous inasmuch as you expose yourself to infection and can cause bleeding that cannot easily be stopped. If you have diabetes or poor circulation, gangrene might follow the self-treatment and eventually cause the loss of the limb or even of life itself.

Only when it is impossible to visit a podiatrist should you ever attempt superficial cutting of the dead skin of the corn. Even then, you must remember that you are practicing "bathroom surgery," which could be dangerous if you aren't careful. Before you do any cutting, first wash your corn and the area around it with soap and warm water, dry it, and then moisten it with an antiseptic, either peroxide or alcohol. Sterilize a sharp knife or razor blade, or even a small sharp scissors, with the same antiseptic solution, and use the sterilized instrument to snip off the top of the corn. Remove only a small portion of the dead, horny skin. Beware not to cut deeply into the corn. If you do, you might cut

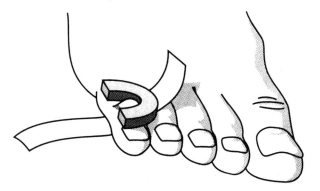

Figure 6.6
To pad a hard corn, place moleskin or podiatry felt, one-eighth to one-quarter of an inch thick, around the corn, and affix with adhesive tape. To reduce inflammation, add a dab of soothing cream into the cutout hole.

into living tissue, and the problem likely would become far more serious than the corn ever was.

Cutting open a shoe to relieve pressure on a corn sometimes gains quick relief from the pain. For corns on the small toe, take off the shoe, then cut along the side at the point where the upper meets the sole. That will relieve the pressure on the top of the toe, and the pain will diminish. Don't be concerned how the shoe might look right now; such a cut in the shoe might not readily be noticed.

Treating a corn with commercial corn plasters probably should be avoided. Corn plasters contain an acid that can burn healthy skin as easily as it will burn dead skin. And a simple corn incorrectly treated with corn plasters can easily become ulcerated.

To treat the soft corns, which form between the toes, you have only to keep the toes separated. To do that most effectively, use lamb's wool or cotton. A small felt pad, like those used for hard corns, can also be employed for that purpose.

A corn at the tip of the toe can result from wearing shoes that are too small or from a slight contracture of the toe. Either can cause the tip of the toe to hammer—to strike against the insole—at every step. Lifting the tip of the toe with adhesive tape halts the hammering. It's good self-help. Once the hammering has stopped, the corn will disappear.

Balancing the foot is also a means of removing corns. With the help of an arch lift or of a corrective series of strappings and paddings, the balance of the foot can be altered, and the pressure on the painful corn can be relieved. The new balance will remove the friction, and the corn possibly will disappear. Arch supports and other foot-balancing appliances provide ways for podiatrists to attempt to correct foot disabilities without resorting to surgery.

TEMPORARY CARE FROM THE PODIATRIST

If you consult a foot doctor to receive temporary corn relief, the usual palliative procedure will be to cut off the upper layers of the uncomfortable corn and to pick out the central area with a pointed instrument. Usually, there is no pain with that treatment, and you get excellent relief—until the skin resumes its growth and becomes so thick that it has to be cut off again. Skin regrowth might take place within one to six weeks.

The podiatrist can also remove corns with a controlled cauterizing ointment. To peel horny skin painlessly and conveniently, although somewhat less quickly, he applies the ointment periodically for a few weeks. The average corn is slowly eliminated by the cauterizing treatment. The podiatrist then fits the toe with a thin, washable, removable, rubber toe shield to keep the corn from returning. This non-surgical treatment succeeds only if the patient wears his or her toe shield constantly.

Palliation is a good and useful treatment. It offers immediate relief for the patient and is rendered at a reasonable fee, but it won't be reimbursed by health insurance policies, which often cover surgical correction. Also, rubber toe shields, foot-balancing appliances, and arch supports are seldom, if ever, compensated for by the health insurance carrier. Orthotic devices are categorized with eyeglasses.

CORN CURES THROUGH MINIMAL-INCISION SURGERY

Corns of all six types are easily corrected permanently by ambulatory foot surgery using minimal-incision techniques. Those easy procedures often involve less time to perform than other types of surgery. Very little follow-up care is required. The recovery period is short. The healed part looks and feels as if no operation had taken place there.

Perhaps best of all, the surgery site undergoes very little injury. Complete correction on the operating table allows the patient to walk—figuratively speaking—from the clinic's operating table to the factory workbench. If there should be any postoperative discomfort, it will usually occur only along the minimal incision. Therefore, when a patient has ambulatory foot surgery, he or she can expect to be free of pain permanently from the moment a local anesthetic is administered.

7. *All About Bunions*

THERE are two types of bunions. The acute bunion causes the sharper pain. It develops from a bursitis, a sudden outcropping of a fluid-filled sac. The acute bunion can progress into the second type of bunion, the hallux valgus, a chronic but often painless deformity involving permanent rigidity of the bones. (See Figure 7.1.)

Bunions can form in any part of the foot but occur most often at the big toe joint, where the first metatarsal bone abuts the proximal phalanx of the big toe. Women are more likely than men to get bunions, because of the misshapen footgear and elevated heels they wear.

DIRECT CAUSE OF BUNIONS

Bursitis is an inflammation of a bursa, which is a sac containing tissue fluid about the consistency of an egg white. The bursa at the big toe joint acts as a lubricant between the skin and the bones. Continual irritation of the skin by an ill-fitting shoe causes the sac to become inflamed and inflated with more fluid. When that occurs, the condition is an acute and painful bursitis.

During the early phases of bursitis, the fluid tries to force itself to the surface of the skin so that it can be discharged. There is minimal but continuous irritation at the joint. If you ignore the irritation, hardening of the skin takes place. The forward displacement that occurs when your foot is fitted into high-heeled shoes, or even into stockings that are

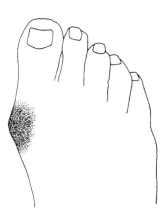

Figure 7.1
Although some redness is present on the top of the distorted big toe joint, the hallux valgus bunion does not hurt this foot.

too snug, adds to the pressures upon the joint. The bursal fluid begins to solidify into a mass that resembles gelatin. The result will be a bunion joint, which then enters a subacute phase.

At this point, you can still prevent a painful, unsightly foot deformity. If, however, either from a lack of information or from fashion vanity you allow it to progress, the condition will grow worse. It does so because the bunion makes one's task of finding a properly fitted shoe even more difficult. A high-heeled shoe, if it is to stay on your foot, must fit snugly at the heel. The shoe salesperson might give you a snug heel fit, all right, but he or she usually does it by fitting you—or by allowing you to fit yourself—with shoes that are too small. By this time, the ball of your foot, with its bulbous outcropping of bunion, is considerably wider than the heel. The shoe with a snug heel that prevents slippage at its back might not fit the normal width of the ball of the foot at the front of the shoe. Indeed, with the added growth of bunion, the width of the foot can no longer be considered normal. Thus, the improper fit at the ball of the foot leads to an angulation of the big toe joint. This deformity is a hallux valgus.

HALLUX VALGUS

The American Podiatry Association, curious about the incidence of bunions in women, conducted a survey of 218 female patients age 40 and over. The survey confirmed that hallux valgus is a common affliction. Every one of the women had the condition in either a mild or severe form, ranging from inflammation to bone deformity to invalidism.

Podiatrists agree that hallux valgus is a serious condition. It strains the foot and produces an abnormal prominence of the joints; it also widens the front of the foot and causes a loss of balance. And any deformation of the big toe interferes with standing and walking. Then, too, malposition of the big toe bone and loss of power in the foot muscles can lead early in life to arthritis.

As hallux valgus progresses, the tendons of the toes shorten, the muscles contract, and all the bones in the front of the foot are displaced. Continued wearing of pointed-toe shoes creates an even greater angulation of the bones at the front of the foot. The ligaments and the joint capsules adapt to the changed position. Because there is no pain, it is not uncommon for little or no attention to be given to the problem. Only the ugliness of the feet is bothersome. Most persons who have bunions will do nothing about it, because there is no pain to draw attention to the deformity steadily taking place.

You can still prevent those deformed feet from becoming more misshapen. Try to eliminate any pressure from shoes and stockings.

You might pad the foot with felt or rubber to minimize stresses on the joint. If suitable attention is not given to the abnormality at this time, a true crippling probably will take place.

Bony spurs can form on either side of the big toe bone and metatarsal head, and the constant friction at the joint angle can cause calcification at the points of stress. The first metatarsal muscle becomes so weak and wasted that it loses its ability to move the toe. The foot fans out in front. The small sesamoid bones under the first metatarsal are deflected. Finally, the big toe angulates more and, ultimately, lies across or under the second toe. In that way, hallux valgus can lead to another problem: hammertoe.

FOOT FACT

Foot problems occur four times more often in women than in men.

If you have allowed the bunion to be aggravated to this point before you have reached middle age, then the joint will probably start to hurt again when you are in your fifties. Then, however, the pain might not come from bursitis, but from osteoarthritis or from corns and calluses that form at the site of friction and pressure. The expansion of the joint might become permanent. In that case, the deformity can be accommodated only by bigger shoes and by rubber toe shields. Shoe linings opposite the joint can tear, further aggravating the problem.

There is a shoe of unusual depth—the bunion-last shoe—that will accommodate a foot that has a bunion at the big toe. The upper of the shoe is fitted with extra leather around the instep. It is deep and has extra width in the front to accommodate bunions. Most orthopedic shoe stores offer such shoes.

Although you are not born with bunions, you can be disposed genetically to their development. Certain foot shapes are more likely than others to develop bunions. Podiatrists state that bunions can be genetically traced in thirty percent of the patients who have them. Thus, if you have a long big toe, it might deform more easily since, when you walk, greater leverage is exerted upon it.

People who must stand in one place for many hours can strain their feet. That strain is likely to produce a bunion. An infection in the big toe joint can also weaken the joint and lead to hallux valgus.

Certain natives of Africa such as the Sambuci, who have never worn shoes, develop hallux valgus, apparently because of a hereditary or congenital tendency. It is likely, however, that those particular feet were injured at some time and that an inflammation gave rise to the deformity.

NON-SURGICAL RELIEF FROM BUNIONS

Podiatric medicine has methods of relief and correction for bunions. In one non-surgical treatment, the joint is stretched by a traction machine.

The traction reduces the adhesions and so alleviates the pain. The machine may incorporate oscillation (concentrated vibration). Cortisone injected directly into the joint will reduce inflammation, but it actually causes a dissolution of the joint and is not recommended.

The best injection procedure available for bunion correction is known as reconstructive therapy. A homeopathic remedy or a sclerotherapeutic agent is injected to irritate the ligaments surrounding the joint so that they grow stronger and firmer.

A bunion deformity develops because of overstretching of ligaments on the inner border of the big toe joint and contraction of the ligaments on the outer border. For permanent correction, the ligaments have to be treated. This is done either by injection or by minimal-incision surgery. Whichever procedure is done for your bunion problem, correction is assured. You don't have to suffer.

HELPING YOURSELF

The podiatrist is aware that narrow, pointed-toe shoes provide insufficient space for toe movement and are the major cause of bunions. The feet are not rigid; they must flex, bend, and move. But women seldom wear shoes with enough room in the toes to allow forward extension of the feet when standing or with enough room for expansion of the feet when walking.

Feet lengthen with normal use. When tired, they expand more—they might even swell. As time goes by, the expansion becomes permanent. You might be wearing a shoe today that is one or two sizes larger than the shoe you wore ten years ago. For that reason, it is important that you insist upon proper measurement of your feet every time you buy a pair of shoes. It is foolhardy to insist upon buying shoes in a particular size just because you have worn that size for years. If your foot has grown longer and is held in a pointed-toe shoe in your previous shoe size, then pressure from the shoe will exert a powerful, concentrated, deflecting force on the toes and could even dislocate them. Many pounds of pressure are exerted on the foot as you take a step. The force of this pressure causes bunions.

No matter how much money you spend, a shoe fit is only as good as the salesperson who does the fitting. If you suffer from bunions, do not allow yourself to be misfitted. Try on long, wide shoes created from lasts that combine a narrow heel and a wide forepart. If the shoe that fits at the toe is too wide at the heel, the shoe salesperson can strategically shrink it with a hot, moist iron or can tighten it with non-slip pads.

Shoes, so comfortable when they are right for you, can be harmful if they are wrong for the shape of your feet. The danger from a crippling

How to Correct Bunions With a Can of Campbell's Soup

Nothing is more welcome to the bunion sufferer than a viable method of correcting the ugly and misshapen protuberance without resorting to surgery. The following self-help procedure, when practiced faithfully each day for at least one hour, might do some straightening of the bunion deformation:

1. Soak the feet for fifteen minutes in a warm Epsom salt solution deep enough to cover both feet entirely to just under the anklebones.
2. Dry them thoroughly with a Turkish towel.
3. Sit on a low chair or stool with your feet bare and still warm from the foot bath. Have on hand a sealed metal can that is 4 inches high, 2½ inches in diameter, and filled with food–Campbell's Condensed Vegetarian Vegetable Soup fills the need admirably.
4. Loop a sturdy, inch-wide rubber band (preferably six inches in circumference) over the forward phalanges of both big toes.
5. With your feet held together at the two big toes by the rubber band, slip the Campbell's soup can between your arches. The heels will be apart and will stick out in back. The can should stand upright.
6. Move your heels together so that the big toes are stretched apart by the rubber band joining them. (For greater traction on the toes, reach down and push your heels even closer together.)
7. Hold that position as long as possible, relaxing the tension only when unendurable pain is created in the big toe muscles.
8. Perform this exercise each day for an hour or more. It may take as long as half a year to see progress in correcting your bunion deformity.
9. When you are through with the exercise, reward yourself by opening the can, pouring its contents into a pot, warming it on the stove, and eating the soup.

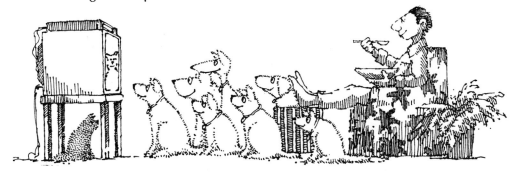

deformity such as a bunion is not to be dismissed lightly. Ask anybody who has ever suffered from one.

PERMANENTLY CORRECTING BUNIONS

Bunions are a serious matter. They strain the feet and eventually can bring on arthritis, manifested in the outgrowth of bony spurs on either side of the big toe joints. The only true correction is bunion surgery, but surgery through large open wounds immobilizes the patient for weeks after his leaving the hospital. The open-wound operation can involve a three- to six-inch incision for the removal of the sesamoid bones, the lengthening of the tendons, the removal of a wedge of bone from the metatarsal, and the excision of arthritic spurs that produce bony bulges. At the same time, the joint capsule is cut, and the remaining structures might be wired in place. The open-wound procedure is still being used in about half the bunionectomies performed today, despite advances made in the past generation.

In 1963, Dr. J.N. Wilson, an English orthopedic surgeon, developed an improved bunion surgery technique. Modification of the Wilson procedure soon thereafter made bunion removal in the podiatry office a common occurrence. The modification was perfected by podiatrist Seymour Kessler, a founder and past president of the Academy of Ambulatory Foot Surgeons. The Kessler operation has been adopted as the standard for bunion operations performed by minimal-incision surgeons. Using local anesthesia, the surgeon makes an incision smaller than one-half inch and removes part of the bony protuberance. Following surgery, the large toe is repositioned and held in place with a sturdy adhesive-tape dressing, which is worn for about three weeks. Complete healing takes place in six to eight weeks, and patients require no more than a mild prescription sedative for any discomfort.

Dr. Kessler has said, "We use a special surgical instrument that resembles the drill used in dentistry. The conventional surgical knife, hammer, and mallet are not employed to cut away growths. Instead, protuberances are removed by our new surgical tool to the point that the operated area can quickly and clearly be realigned. Artificial support implants (such as pins, wires, and staples) to allow the severed bones to knit in their new positions are unnecessary."

The Kessler bunion technique relies on the patient's own intact skin and muscle to provide a natural support, implemented by bandaging and taping. The patient leaves the ambulatory foot surgeon's office wearing a surgical shoe instead of a cast. Most people who undergo the minimal-incision method return to work the next day. This holistic foot procedure reduces the risk of infection.

FINANCIAL EDGE

The bill for traditional bunion surgery performed in the hospital is nearly $10,000. But when the operation is done in the foot doctor's office, the bill is about only one-tenth of that amount.

Health insurance policies pay for both types of bunionectomy. "At one time," said Garry Garrison, an official with Blue Cross/Blue Shield, "a patient needed a rider on his health insurance policy to be covered for outpatient care. Now we'll pay whether the surgery is outpatient or inpatient." This revised philosophy is encouraging a movement in health care away from the hospital to an increased use of the doctor's office as a surgical suite.

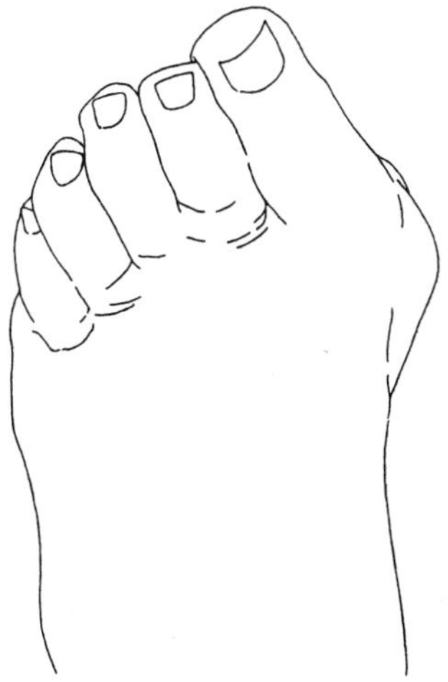

A TALE OF TWO BUNIONECTOMIES

After reading about ambulatory foot surgery in her husband's service club magazine, Dorothea H., age 54, contacted the national office of the Academy of Ambulatory Foot Surgeons for referral to a podiatrist for minimal-incision surgery on her bunion. The ambulatory surgeon evaluated the bunion and learned that the woman was anxious to get rid of the unsightly protuberance on her big toe joint.

It was not a huge bunion, but it was large enough to make Dorothea feel that it detracted from her appearance when she went barefoot in public such as at the local swimming pool. The bunion was surgically removed. During her entire recuperative period of a few months, Dorothea experienced practically no discomfort. She now has no bunion and no scar from the minimal incision. (See Figures 7.2 and 7.3.)

Trying to rid herself of a bunion that was exceedingly painful, Virginia I., age 60, sought relief. A podiatrist applied palliative measures, but the pain continued. The woman stated her wish to have the bunion removed permanently. The podiatrist obliged her. She had lived with her foot problem for more than thirty years, and now it was gone forever by means of a minimal-incision bunionectomy. (See Figures 7.4 and 7.5.)

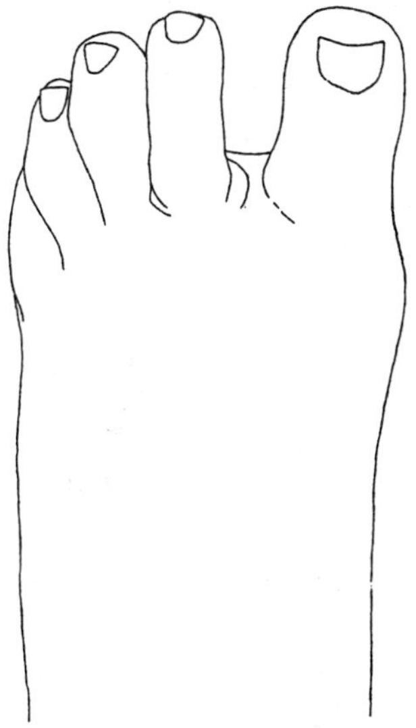

CORRECTING ROSALYN D.'S BUNIONS

When 46-year-old Rosalyn D. read her hometown newspaper on July 8, 1984, she saw a story about a relatively new treatment for foot problems which utilized power equipment similar to a dentist's drill. Surgery performed by an ambulatory foot surgeon, wrote the reporter,

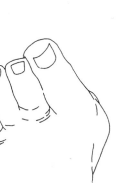

Figure 7.2
An artist's rendering of the unsightly bunion of Dorothea H., before surgery.

Figure 7.3
Four months later, Dorothea's bunion has been removed by minimal-incision surgery.

usually allows patients to walk out of the doctor's office on their own and with their foot problems permanently eliminated.

The article vitally interested Rosalyn, since she recognized her desire for office-based, minimal-incision, ambulatory foot surgery. For much of her adult life she had suffered, first with acute and then chronic bunions on both her feet.

She had once had an acute bunion on the foot where the first metatarsal bone meets the big toe. It was bursitis, a painfully swollen sac containing fluid. Since the inflamed bursa was not treated, the tissues hardened. The condition worsened, and an angulation of the big toe joint set in. Over an extended period, this angulation turned into a chronic bunion. Rosalyn now had a true bone deformity, a hallux valgus.

"The only true correction is bunion surgery," an orthopedic surgeon had told her twelve years earlier. He had described how she would require hospitalization for the straightening of her big toes, the chopping off of her two bulbous bunion joints with a mallet and chisel, and the repositioning of her metatarsal bones. Into each foot the orthopedist intended to make a two-inch incision between the first and second metatarsal bones. Plus, a huge half-moon incision would start at the bottom front portion of each big toe and would extend well up on the inner longitudinal arch past the bunion area. The latter incision would be more than four inches in length and would act as the entry point for the hallux valgus correction.

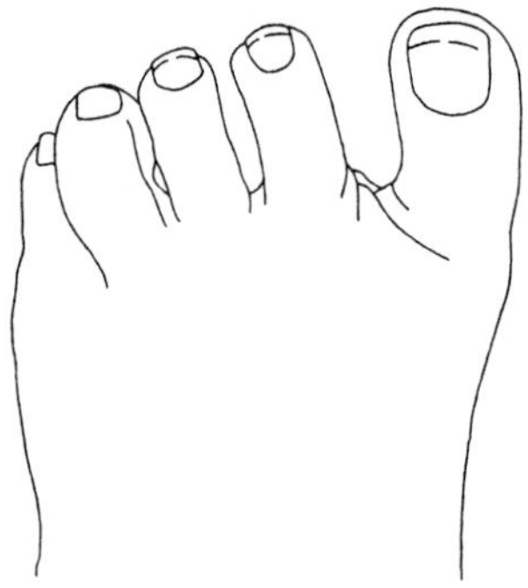

The orthopedic surgeon's operative technique would require Rosayln to stay five days in the hospital, then three weeks in bed at home. She could return to work only after waiting out six weeks of recuperation time—and then only after switching to a job that would keep her off her feet. She probably would need to use crutches for three months to hobble from place to place. When Rosalyn asked the orthopedist if the standard bunion procedure he was proposing would hurt, the answer was a simple but honest yes!

Is it any wonder that Rosalyn D. decided against having bunion surgery? For twelve years, she had accepted bunion discomfort as part of living. Now, that's all changed. Her bunions are permanently gone.

"I read the story about minimal-incision ambulatory foot surgery that's performed in the office. It was obvious that this was the way I wanted to be treated," said Rosalyn. "I visited the podiatry office of an ambulatory foot surgeon. He examined my feet, took X-ray films of them, did laboratory work, and fully explained what had happened. He explained why I had bunions, how they had gradually developed, and how they could be corrected without resorting to the terrible procedures previously described to me. I became fully informed and consented to undergo minimal-incision ambulatory foot surgery. The whole thing was a joy to me.

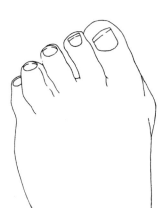

Figure 7.4
An artist's rendering of the foot of Virginia I. before she underwent minimal-incision surgery for removal of an uncomfortable bunion.

Figure 7.5
Two months later, after a minimal-incision bunionectomy, Virginia's foot looked and felt much healthier.

"My right foot was operated on on July 20, 1984, and the left foot was done two weeks later. My bunions were taken off without my feeling any discomfort. Because I had always suffered with painful calluses on the bottoms of my feet, the doctor lifted the first, second, and third metatarsals. Now the calluses also have disappeared. Crooked second toes were straightened, as well. I'm so happy!

"From my use of a small amount of pain medication that was prescribed by the podiatrist, I didn't lose a single night of sleep. I spent no daytime in bed. By mid-August I was moving around well and needed no crutches. I returned to work as a cashier and stood behind the cash register like always. I had no trouble. The whole thing was quick, easy, comfortable, and had me take off from work less than a week. I may not even have required that length of time to recuperate, but I thought I'd give myself the luxury of lounging around the house. Besides, I had a lot of vacation time due me."

8. *Hammertoes: Deformities That Hurt*

HAMMERTOES, one of the most painful of foot ailments, can be traced directly to the wearing of narrow, pointed-toe shoes so typical of contemporary footgear, especially women's. Women most often are the victims of hammertoes. Most of the time, female footwear is not much wider at the front than at the heel. But the ball of a human foot is almost twice as wide as the heel, and the outline of the normal foot is rounded. The combination of narrow shoe and wide foot, of pointed shoe and rounded foot, causes, predictably enough, painful foot problems such as hammertoes.

HAMMERTOE FORMATION

A hammertoe is marked by contracture of the tendons, laxity of the ligaments, and angulation of the second and third phalanges of the toe. The shoes compress the feet and constrict the muscles that move the toes. Subsequently, the muscles waste away, and the motions of the toes become puny and weak. At the same time, the toe is deprived of the room it needs to function effectively.

In all ill-fitting shoe, the toe seeks room anywhere it can be found. The pressure on the sides of the toes, as they are squeezed together by narrow footgear, causes a toe to "hammer." It curls up. It arches until the toenail is nearly vertical. As the pressure continues, the affected toe—the second or third, and sometimes both—might rise, contract, and overlap other toes. (Occasionally, it will underlap other toes.) It's not uncommon for a hammertoe to move up and out of the line of toes and become an extracurricular digit that serves no purpose. It just lays in its pathological state on top of one or more of the other four toes, practically having become a vestigal appendage. (See Figure 8.1.)

The tip of a hammertoe can strike the ground with a thud at every step and become flat and squat. A hard corn can form on top, and a distal corn can form at the hammering portion. The nail might split or grow inward. A corn or callused nail groove might develop where the flesh is caught between the nail and the toe bone or where the toe is angulated. A soft corn can prove especially annoying when it's between the hammertoe and the adjacent toe that is overlapped.

Although any toe may be affected, the second toe suffers most often. It is longer than the other toes and therefore more likely to be deformed by small footgear.

The effects of a hammertoe are not limited to the toe. The toe bones, forced back against the metatarsals, exert pressure against the center of the foot. The ball of the foot suffers, calluses form, and muscular cramps develop.

Wearing tight-fitting stockings, short footgear, tapered-toe shoes, pointed-toe shoes, tight leotards, or really snug pantyhose for long periods of time can produce a hammertoe. Because those items of apparel are necessarily worn on both feet, there can be two hammertoes, one on each foot. Although some people are born with a hereditary contracture, and some acquire a contracture from having a systemic disease such as arthritis, the only thing that increases any hammering tendency from familial or hereditary traits is abuse of the feet from ill-fitting or ill-shaped footgear. Hammering will not occur unless abusive shoes are worn. Some doctors deny this, but they are only fooling themselves if they believe that hammertoe sufferers are born with tendencies for hammertoes.

PALLIATIVE TREATMENT FOR HAMMERTOES

You can try treating a hammertoe on your own with exercise and mechanical stretching. Podiatrists are uncertain as to the value of stretching and exercising to relieve the condition. And only in minor cases do foot doctors attempt manipulation and splinting; even then, many months might pass before even the mildest case responds. Yet, when your own toe is affected, you are willing to try anything, right? Exercising and stretching and the wearing of rubber splints are things you can do for yourself. (See exercises in chapter twenty.)

Attach a small spoon-shaped splint to the hammertoe with a rubber band. Wear the splint during the day and a toe-stretching device at

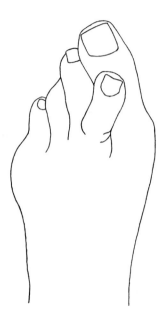

Figure 8.1
This foot sports a useless second toe. The hammertoe sticks up and out of the normal line of toes as if it is a vestigal appendage. It painfully lies across the big toe and makes it decidedly difficult for the foot to be fitted with proper shoes.

night. After a short period, you might impatiently try some other device as a toe support. In the end, your attempt to straighten the toe might be abandoned as you resign yourself to live with the pain.

For temporary relief, lightly tape the protruding toe to hold it down, straight and even with the other toes. Then use tape to create a sling for pulling the offending digit back into normal alignment.

Traction and oscillation, a palliative technique used together on bunions, also applies to hammertoes. A podiatrist runs the machinery. Overall, traction and oscillation is a good but conservative way to manage the condition.

Of course, wearing shoes that fit properly is the best way to avoid hammertoes.

SURGICAL CORRECTION OF HAMMERTOES

Although nothing stops you from first trying home care, treatment by a foot surgeon is probably the best way to deal with a hammertoe.

The podiatrist employing minimal-incision techniques does not remove the toe; instead, he or she uses a power-driven tool to file away a small wedge of bone from the angle of the contracture. The procedure, painless under local anesthetic, takes only a few minutes in the doctor's office. The patient is usually able to walk home but will require a few days to recuperate. The toe is held in its corrected position by a small splint until fusion of the bone takes place, usually within a few weeks.

In an alternative minimal-incision procedure, the foot surgeon lengthens the tendon. Eliminating the contracture of the tendons on the top of the foot strengthens the movement of the hammertoe so it can uncurl and straighten.

Ambulatory foot surgery for correcting hammertoes is not uncomfortable for the patient and not difficult for the foot doctor skilled in the methods of minimal-incision foot surgery. Indeed, this treatment requires only a slight puncture in the skin and no bed confinement.

Thus, hammertoe surgical correction is typical of other minimal-incision ambulatory surgical procedures carried out in the podiatrist's office. It begins with an anesthetic nerve block that numbs the affected area. The foot is scrubbed, then draped with sterile linen. When the anesthetic takes effect, the operation commences.

FOOT FACT

For two out of every ten people, the second toe is the longest.

A HAMMERTOE CASE HISTORY

Mary P., 46 years old, was motivated to correct her hammertoe both for cosmetic and comfort reasons. She felt embarrassed by the distorted

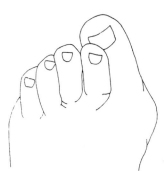

Figure 8.2
An artist's rendering
of the hammertoe and
accompanying bunion
on Mary P.'s left foot.

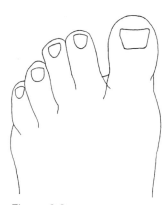

Figure 8.3
Two months later, after
Mary P. underwent minimal-
incision surgery, the double
pathology is gone
permanently.

appearance of her feet, and her big toe was cramped in her high-style footwear. The hammertoe foot had a bunion, too.

She paid a visit to a foot surgeon to learn how her hammertoe could be straightened. The ramifications of all possible treatments were explained to Mary, who then went to an orthopedic surgeon for a second opinion. The orthopedist wanted to remove the involved toe joint, chop off the bunion, and leave her hospitalized for two weeks. Mary opposed such treatment. She realized that, by comparison, ambulatory foot surgery for hammertoe correction is less radical, preserves the integrity of the toe joints, and avoids the unnecessary elimination of joints when the toes must be reset in more desirable positions.

Unlike the holistic approach, the orthopedic surgeon's method had figuratively isolated the woman's toe from the rest of the foot and failed to take into account her whole personhood. With traditional surgery, she would have been laid up with pain for a month after the hospitalization.

Instead, Mary returned to the podiatrist and underwent minimal-incision ambulatory foot surgery. She had her bunion corrected, as well. (See Figures 8.2 and 8.3.) The procedure was quick, painless, and required no bed confinement. She could walk during the entire recuperative period. Two months after her hammertoe straightening, Mary enjoyed a Caribbean cruise during which she comfortably danced in high-heeled pumps.

9. *The Burning Pain of Calluses*

THE pain of calluses demand special measures. That's because calluses bring on an acutely irritating pain that could be described as biting, stinging, smarting, and tormenting, but most especially as burning. The burning pain of calluses is ever present. Each time you take a step, the burn is there, reminding you that all is not happy and healthy on the ball of your foot or along the sides of your big toe.

A callus is a thickened mass of skin that forms on the weight-bearing surfaces of the body. It is caused by constant friction and pressure. A healthy callus forms a natural barrier to objects that can penetrate the skin and damage the sensitive underlying tissues of the body.

Calluses on the hands are usual—so much so that calluses in specific areas can even indicate the kind of work one does. A guitarist, for example, will have calluses at the tips of the fingers on the left hand. Leather tanners, who use their hands to smooth and stretch leather, develop calluses on the heels of their palms. Karate experts deliberately develop massive calluses along the fifth metacarpal (the bone leading from the wrist to the pinky). There are calluses on the palms of woodcutters and other manual workers. When the calluses are no longer needed to protect the flesh, as when the woodcutter retires or abandons his work, the healthy callus can soften and peel off.

Even on the feet, calluses are not unusual. The natives of New Guinea and the aborigines in Australia can have tough calluses on the soles of their feet. Those calluses are normal and protect the soles from the ground upon which the bare feet move.

The burning calluses we are speaking of, however, have no semblance of healthiness to them. They grow thick, encrusted, and abnormal in places they don't belong, such as at the borders of the big toe where it gets pinched inside the shoe between the insole and the upper. (See Figure 9.1.) This type of unhealthy callus burns; the burning is a sign that the callus contains the seeds of pathology.

PATHOLOGICAL CALLUS

Pathological calluses grow on the bottom of the feet where the weight-bearing pressures of the body are concentrated. These pathological entities are hard, dry, horn-like masses of yellowish or grayish skin that vary in size. They are thick in the center and gradually taper at the sides. Each can have a deep, hard, gray central area like a corn has. Because the thickened skin loses its elasticity and no longer stretches to normal length across the ball of the foot when the feet are flexed, these calluses burn with a fury.

Faulty weight distribution frequently leads to the formation of calluses. Tight footgear can compress the foot and cause a metatarsal bone to be displaced—that is, to drop below the other metatarsals. Should that occur, the foot will function abnormally. The weight of the body would be badly distributed and be borne on only one bone—the dropped metatarsal—at any moment in the natural stride. With all the weight of the body pressing down on an area the size of a pinhead (the bottoms of some metatarsal bones come to a point), the skin, caught between the bone above and the sole below, is killed. The dead skin accumulates and forms a conical structure with its apex turned inward into the foot, thus creating a kind of corn, and the callus spreads outward. When one metatarsal bone carries excessive weight, the ligaments that hold the bones together become overstretched, and another metatarsal bone might drop. Eventually, the entire metatarsal arch can collapse.

The callus formed by the dropped metatarsal, painful as it is, is not in itself important. It is only a sign that something else is wrong—the dropped metatarsal. Treatment of such a foot problem must be directed not at the callus, which is a result, but at the fallen anterior metatarsal arch, which is the cause and needs to be restored.

CALLUSES FROM HIGH-HEELED SHOES

High-heeled shoes are a major cause of calluses' developing on the balls of the feet. The body's weight should be distributed throughout the foot, from the heel forward, but high-heeled shoes shift the weight to

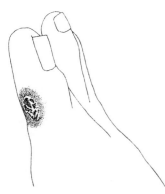

Figure 9.1
A callus is liable to grow at the lower border of the big toe if skin is pinched in the shoe between the upper and the insole.

the metatarsals. The ball of the foot then takes on the function of the heel, and thick skin soon develops.

At first, the thick skin forms primarily to protect the foot. But as the thickening continues and the skin loses elasticity, there is an awful burning sensation. The burning compels the sufferer to avoid applying pressure. New changes in weight distribution take place, new areas of stress develop, and severe foot fatigue follows.

Calluses can also come from chronic skin conditions such as eczema, psoriasis, and fungus infections, and from systemic diseases such as thyroid malfunction. Poor blood circulation and diabetes, both systemic disorders, can each turn an ordinary callus into a deep, weeping ulcer.

SELF-TREATMENT FOR CALLUSES

To get relief from calluses, it is important to spread the weight evenly over the entire ball of the foot. That can be accomplished by padding the callus with shock-absorbing material, such as felt or foam rubber. Apply it directly onto the skin around the uncomfortable spot. The padding, properly pared, is fitted on both sides and behind the callus to remove the weight completely from the affected location. (See Figure 9.2.)

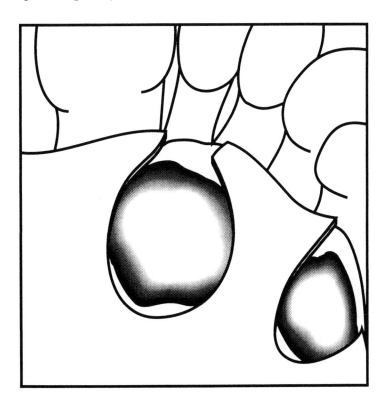

Figure 9.2
Cutout felt pads conforming in shape to calluses on the bottom of a foot and skived at the edges can be placed around the calluses to take the pressure off them and relieve the pain.

Attention should also be given to the shoes. They must be wide enough for the foot to expand to its full width without being crowded. If the shoes are too narrow, they have to be replaced at once with wider footgear.

If your callus has become thick and bothersome, it must be softened. Soak the foot in a solution of bicarbonate of soda or in a one percent solution of potassium hydroxide. A warm soapy foot bath might also help. When the callus has softened sufficiently, the thickened skin can be rubbed away with a pumice stone or a rough Turkish towel.

Calluses will return week after week, however, unless the pressure and weight that cause them are removed from the dropped metatarsal. A cutout felt pad works well for that purpose. Store-bought arch supports rarely do the job. Even molded shoes are not the final solution. Only a foot-molded appliance will provide permanent help.

FOOT-MOLDED APPLIANCES AND OTHER CALLUS CARE

To distribute weight evenly on the sole of the foot, the podiatrist can make a pair of orthopedic foot appliances that will fit easily into the shoes or onto the feet. The appliances are called *orthotics,* balancing devices worn under the feet inside the shoes. They will likely be made from a cast or imprint of the feet. The appliances transfer the body's weight to non-callused areas and allow the callused area to float with no weight pressing on it.

Most podiatrists can make a foot-shaped pad that will be worn in the shoe under the lining or between the bare foot and the sock. The use of such a pad is generally successful at relieving and even preventing calluses.

The podiatrist can apply a softening ointment that removes the callus easily. He continues the treatment with moleskin padding, placing the pad not on top of the callus but around it or behind it. The pad takes the pressure off the callus.

The doctor might also advise placing a bar of leather on the outside of the shoe across the ball of the sole. The shoemaker calls that an anterior heel or metatarsal bar. It works like a foot pad but is not quite as effective.

The object of using orthopedic modalities is to prevent the skin from being caught between the dropped metatarsal bone above and the shoe sole below. Such excessive pressure kills the skin, causing accumulation in thickened layers and producing a conical structure that grows inwardly, resulting in pain with every step. If the conical structure remains, it probably should be removed surgically.

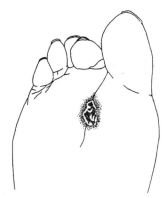

Figure 9.3
An artist's rendering of Mary B.'s right foot. Her high arch made her metatarsals drop. Three calluses formed under the sole of her foot. The deeply grown one under her second metatarsal area burned with every step, and the others didn't feel so good, either.

SURGICAL TREATMENT FOR CALLUSES

The metatarsal bones on Mary B.'s right foot had dropped as a result of her extremely high-arched feet. Inevitably, she developed calluses. (See Figure 9.3.) She needed major reconstruction. Ordinary orthopedic surgery would have kept her out of work for three months. Orthopedic procedures for foot reconstruction usually require inserting metal pins, applying casts, and having the patient use crutches to get around. Instead, Mary underwent a series of minimal-incision procedures to raise her metatarsal bones and straighten an associated underlapping hammertoe. (See Figure 9.4.) During the entire recuperative period, she continued her hobby of teaching dance three nights a week, and she never remained home from work. It was important for her to maintain those activities.

When last checked on, years after the minimal-incision operation, Mary continued to have no callus pain and to keep up her teaching of dance.

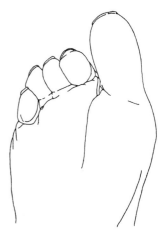

Figure 9.4
Following an operation using minimal-incision surgery, Mary is free of pain. Her three calluses are practically entirely gone, in particular the one that had burned under her second metatarsal. Her hammertoe was straightened, too.

10. *Finding the Cure for Foot Warts*

DOESN'T everyone recognize warts? They're small excrescences of flesh that grow on your hands after you've picked up a toad. Right?

No! That amusing bit of folklore is acknowledged by most of us—some little boys excepted—to be a superstition. That, however, is the extent of knowledge many people have about warts. (It must be admitted that science can tell us little more about the causes of warts. No wonder the superstition about toads has flourished.)

Warts are, of course, blemishes wherever they appear. Warts can be painful, although frequently they are not. Usually, they are simply annoying. Nevertheless, most people who have warts want to get rid of them. To judge from the number of patients who go to a doctor's office after cutting or treating a wart at home, those excrescences are sufficiently bothersome to be given attention. But anyone who tries to cut a wart has already violated a cardinal rule: Keep your hands off! Never cut into a wart.

Medical science identifies many kinds of warts. Pitch warts are common to workers who handle pitch and coal tar; post-mortem warts occur on the hands of those whose duties require them to make post-mortem dissections; venereal warts appear as the result of gonorrheal or syphilitic infections.

Foot warts are non-cancerous infectious swellings of the skin that can spread from one part of the body to another and from one person to another. They are especially common among children. The majority of foot warts disappear without treatment, but some are persistent and require heroic measures. The two warts known to grow specifically on the feet are the plantar and the mosaic.

PLANTAR WART

A plantar wart, or *verruca plantaris,* is a raised lump of flesh on the sole of the foot. (See Figure 10.1.) It is really a benign tumor that is well supplied with blood vessels and nerves. One might mistake it for a corn or a callus because it is covered with callus tissue and because it hurts. Still, with a little study, you can readily distinguish between corn, callus, and wart.

The surest way to tell a plantar wart from other growths is to pinch it slightly; the excruciating pain that follows will immediately indicate it is a plantar wart. Also, the plantar wart is pearly white, soft, and spongy, with a center that shows tiny spots of black, brown, or red. Those spots are blood vessels that supply the wart with nutrition. Walking flattens the wart so that it remains thickened and rough in texture. Varying in size from a pinhead to a quarter, and usually appearing under the weight-bearing parts of the foot, the plantar wart can grow either singly or in clusters.

MOSAIC WART

An irregular, dry, horny mass of tissue, the mosaic wart often is painless but sometimes gives discomfort of a burning nature. The mosaic wart could be covered by a thick callus and consists of hundreds of little seedlike warts. (See Figure 10.2.) A patch of mosaic warts might vary in size and possibly grow to cover the entire bottom of the foot. The irregular appearance of those patches gives the mosaic wart its name.

The mosaic and plantar varieties usually start as tiny bumps on the skin of the sole of the foot, although they can also form on the thinner skin at the top of a foot. The small bumps gradually become larger, rough-surfaced (especially rough is the mosaic), and brownish. They are likely to appear in conjunction with calluses and become extremely painful when forced inward by the pressure of body weight.

CAUSES OF WARTS

While science cannot tell us exactly why foot warts appear, there is a strong suspicion—even microscopic evidence—that they are caused by

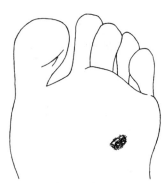

Figure 10.1
This typical plantar wart growing under the fourth metatarsal head is covered with thick callus and contains many tiny blood vessels.

an infection from the human papilloma virus. Yes, a virus causes the tiny tumor—the papilloma—known as a wart. It enters the skin of the foot after a slight injury and takes a foothold in the underlying dermal layers. The virus has an incubation period ranging from three weeks to six months. All warts are spread by scratching or shaving—and in the case of plantar and mosaic warts, by going about barefoot in public places.

The wart virus can be in your shoes, on the floor of a gym or a locker room, in a swimming pool, or wherever else people go barefoot in public. Infected people can leave behind in their footsteps small flakes of skin that attach to your own foot sole and then invade the dermis.

One theory maintains that a foot injury can be a factor in causing foot warts. According to that speculation, the body alters the skin to seal off the irritation or injury. Another theory maintains that warts indicate a disturbance in the blood chemistry or in the endocrine system.

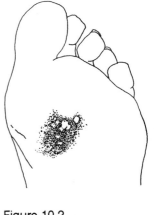

Figure 10.2
A mosaic wart has spread across the first, second, and third metatarsal heads. It is an irregular, dry, horny growth covered with thick callus. It bleeds readily when irritated.

It seems possible that the mosaic wart is, in some way, connected with athlete's foot. In our present and former podiatric practices, we have occasionally isolated fungus organisms in cultures grown from wart tissue; we have also seen warts disappear when patients were treated for athlete's foot.

The podiatrist has his or her wart season. Patients usually appear in the fall after having exposed their bare feet to injury during the summer months. Such injuries do not have to be sudden or acute. The continuous minor agitation that comes from walking long distances over rough country roads in thin-soled shoes might be enough to stimulate the forming of a wart. Walking barefoot on beaches or acquiring a stone bruise seems to cause a wart often. Plantar warts also seem to form frequently on the soles of the feet of some athletes in track, basketball, football, soccer, rugby, tennis, lacrosse, and handball—presumably because of the constant foot friction involved in those sports. Teenagers being more sports-minded than other age groups, it is not surprising that they get warts more often than do adults.

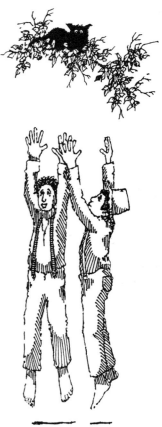

SELF-HELP TREATMENT FOR FOOT WARTS

In *Tom Sawyer*, Huck and Tom planned to remove warts by killing a black cat and burying it at midnight by the light of the full moon. Some believe that one can get rid of warts by rubbing them with castor oil or by tying a bulb of garlic around the victim's neck.

Such superstitious "cures" are ludicrous—that is, until one hears of cases where such cures seemingly have worked. A more likely explanation is that the "cure" has not worked at all but that faith helped solve the wart problem. Science simply does not know what makes a wart appear or disappear. We have heard that psychotherapy has been used to eliminate plantar warts; what actually caused them to go away no one knows.

Although a wart can be uncomfortable, it is not dangerous unless abused. "Bathroom surgery," such as paring a wart down with a razor blade, can lead to an infection; the use of a patent remedy intended for corns might stimulate or irritate the wart and turn it into a dangerous growth. To avoid such dangers, keep all cutting instruments away from plantar warts. Instead, here is how you might get relief:

Cover the foot wart with an astringent cream, which causes it to pucker like a prune. Place a dressing of plastic wrap over the cream, and tape the plastic snugly around the edges to exclude air. Leave the dressing in place for as long as you're willing to stand it, and keep soap and water away from the occluded area. Such treatment has been known to cause the wart tissue to resolve itself, presumably by asphyxiating the aerobic papilloma virus—you have prevented its access to oxygen. The only other answer is to take the problem to your dermatologist or podiatrist.

PODIATRIC ATTENTION FOR FOOT WARTS

Although there are various medical treatments for foot warts, doctors have not found a method that works in every case. A favorite treatment is to cauterize warts with acid. The foot doctor then applies a drug to peel off the warts layer by layer. The acid does not burn; there are many mild acids, similar to ointments, that can remove the warts painlessly. Acid treatments typically take from three to eight weeks, sometimes longer. Such treatments are usually applied to large warts. Throughout the treatment period, one can walk around without pain.

An electric needle can eliminate a wart with a single application. The doctor uses a local anesthetic to numb the wart area and then sparks it out with the needle. After that, about a month is needed for postoperative care. Electric needle treatment is most effective with small warts.

LASER SURGERY

The newest wart removal method is laser therapy. Referred to in medicine as "the scalpel of light," the surgical laser has been used successfully for forty-five years to cut, weld, vaporize, seal, and stimulate healing in human tissue. With a single beam of light brighter than the sun, focused in a straight, narrow, concentration on the foot wart, the laser performs healing miracles. (Laser is an acronym for light amplification by stimulated emission of radiation.)

"Lasers are a mainstay of podiatric surgery," says Barry R. Kaplan, doctor of podiatric medicine and co-director of Arizona Foot Institute Inc. "The laser technique hardly causes discomfort when removing foot warts. But this instrument has to be used by skilled hands."

The laser in wart removal employs a clear carbon dioxide beam, which is absorbed by water. The beam is able to drill a hole through steel but is no match for a wet handkerchief. The moisture in and around human body cells helps ensure safe laser use by diffusing the beam's power. The foot surgeon therefore takes advantage of the high moisture content in cells he or she wants to remove by heating them up and causing them to evaporate. The cells just vanish in a mist of steam. The carbon dioxide in the beam is invisible, but it is tagged with a parallel beam of helium, which produces a red ray to guide the foot surgeon.

Inasmuch as the vaporization occurs so quickly, there is almost no heat transmission to adjacent cells. The area of destruction is strictly confined to where the surgeon is directing the light beam. Laser light is far superior to other forms of thermal destruction, such as the electric needle.

By changing the laser beam's focus, the foot surgeon can either make a scalpel incision or rapidly vaporize tissue in an airbrush fashion. Neither procedure causes damage to adjacent or underlying tissue. Its amazing versatility makes the carbon dioxide laser uniquely valuable for foot surgery.

Following are some of the many advantages of laser surgery for foot warts and some other foot conditions:

- The laser has no blade, so cutting and scarring are held to a minimum.
- Since the beam has a method of cauterizing wounds, bleeding is controlled.
- The laser is self-sterilizing, so the chance for wound infection is almost entirely eliminated. (In fact, the beam penetrates tissue to destroy bacteria and viruses upon contact.)
- Surgical sites once difficult to reach, such as neuromas (nerve tumors), can now be readily contacted and vaporized with a single beam that leaves adjacent tissue relatively unaffected.
- A direct line of sight within the operating area, unobstructed by blood or instruments, is afforded the foot surgeon.
- No dangerous radiation is presented by the laser—certainly no more than that of an ordinary light bulb.
- Clinical studies indicate that foot problems treated with laser surgery have a lower incidence of recurrence.

FOOT FACT

The average foot expands about five percent in volume as the day goes on. It expands much more during extended periods of vigorous exercise.

- Other clinical studies show that nerve endings cut by the carbon dioxide laser are sealed rather than left frayed as by scalpel surgery. (The sealing might account for the decreased postoperative pain noted by patients undergoing laser surgery.)
- With the laser, it is frequently possible to complete in just one visit a treatment that with other techniques might require additional visits or even hospitalization.
- Pregnancy does not preclude the use of the laser beam for surgery. Indeed, the light ray allows for some conditions to receive treatment that otherwise would have to be put off until the pregnancy was over.
- Health insurance companies recognize the benefits of laser surgery; therefore, most laser surgery procedures performed on the foot, such as neuroma removal and permanent excision of toenails, are covered under medical insurance policies.

Laser surgery offers only one disadvantage—a safety risk. But whatever the risk, it falls almost exclusively upon the machine's operator, not on the patient.

OTHER WAYS TO DO AWAY WITH WARTS

Some doctors treat foot warts by freezing them with dry ice. No anesthetic is needed. The patient might, however, find it unpleasant to have a stick of carbon dioxide snow pressed against his foot even for a minute. Yet the treatment works well, especially when given once or twice a week for about six weeks. It can be used in conjunction with the acid treatment.

Newer methods of treating warts also have been developed. Podiatrists, dermatologists, plastic surgeons, and other health professionals sometimes apply solutions that thicken and harden the growths so that they can be peeled out.

Vitamin A has been prescribed. Some authorities believe that a wart develops where there is a lack of vitamin A in the skin and that introducing the vitamin will bring the skin back to normal. An injection that puts vitamin A directly into the warty growth has also been developed.

Orthopedic treatment of warts might help if used in conjunction with another wart removal procedure. The doctor might pad the warty area with soft felt, which can reduce excessive weight at a point on the foot or relieve possible pain by eliminating friction. In time, the wart might disappear of its own accord.

Old-fashioned methods of treating warts can be crude and painful. For example, warts have been burnt out with hot carbon! Radium and

X-rays have also been used against them, but neither is recommended. Both those procedures use radioactive material and pose a danger of altering the skin into a malignant growth.

All the successful and safe treatments described are available if you take your problem to the health professional who treats the skin of the feet. In any case, if you have a foot wart, the only possible way for you to treat yourself safely and effectively is with astringent cream and occlusive dressing. Most home remedies are ineffective if not downright dangerous, for they can lead to foot infection. The best procedure is to regard the wart as a skin tumor and go to a foot or skin specialist. Remember: Keep your hands off all warts—especially warts on the foot.

Part Three

Less-Visible
Foot Problems:
Causes and Treatments

11. *Hot and Itchy Athlete's Foot*

ARE your feet ever hot and itchy? Do you have flaking, peeling, scaling, cracking, or blistering of the skin on the foot soles or between the toes? It is surely no comfort, but if you have those problems you are accompanied by a great many people. Itching feet, with a probable peeling and cracking of the skin and a possible feeling of heat between the toes, are symptoms of athlete's foot, the most common skin malady in the United States today. One pharmaceutical firm that produces an anti-fungal shoe remedy for athlete's foot declares that as many as 80 million Americans—that's nearly one out of three—suffer from the condition. It affects most people in industrialized western countries at some time in their lives.

Actually, "athlete's foot" is a misnomer. The term was first used in the 1920s to designate a particular set of foot symptoms to which men and women who engaged in athletic activities seemed particularly susceptible—and they have been proven susceptible, since they often walk barefoot in shower rooms, locker rooms, and gymnasiums, all of where the condition can easily be transmitted. Yet, athlete's foot is much more widespread than its name would imply. For even in this age of mass participation in sports, there are more persons with athlete's foot than there are athletes.

MULTIPLE CAUSES OF ATHLETE'S FOOT

The medical name for athlete's foot, *tinea pedis*, best describes it and its several causes. Medically, *tinea* means "fungus," and *pedis* means "of the foot." Tinea pedis is not the only cause of athlete's foot, but it is the major one. "Athlete's foot," one must remember, describes the set of symptoms usually manifesting themselves and not the condition's cause. Those symptoms, commonly referred to by the popular name, can also come from allergic reactions to perspiration, drugs, dyes, chemicals, and the like.

Therefore, one of the first tasks of the foot specialist in treating athlete's foot is to identify the source of symptoms as a fungus or an allergy. If a fungus, the answer searched for is which particular microbe must be dealt with; if an allergy, which individual substance in the patient's environment is bringing about an annoying skin reaction of such vast discomfort.

To determine whether a case of athlete's foot is caused by a fungus, the foot doctor scrapes a specimen of skin from the affected area and places it in an agar culture. If a fungus is present on the skin, the culture will grow in a distinctive pattern. The podiatrist might also look at the specimen under a microscope to identify the particular strain of fungus that is responsible for the condition. There are several varieties: *Trichophyton mentagrophytes, Trichophyton rubrum, Epidermophyton floccosum,* and *Candida albicans.* One of those plants is likely to be the cause of the infection.

A fungus by itself does not create a disease. Because the symptom-producing fungus most likely is a parasite, which grows on live tissue (in contrast to a saprophyte, which thrives on dead organic material), it must have a proper medium in which to flourish. The skin on the feet becomes that medium. Much as a toadstool lives and grows in topsoil, the fungus lives and grows on viable skin, thriving best in the skin of corns and calluses. Note that fungi on the skin are ectoparasites living on your body surface, with you being its host. The parasite, which spends nearly all of its existence with the host, obtains food and shelter from the host and contributes nothing to the host's welfare. You get nothing from your athlete's foot, therefore, except foot misery with irritation and an interference of bodily functions.

Although not everyone has accumulations of pathological skin such as corns and calluses, millions of people have conditions favorable to fungus growth on their feet. Those conditions are encouraged by our high-technology existence in a society that has gotten used to the conveniences of life. Even what we eat—the low-quality foods furnished by fast-food restaurants, for instance—is a major cause for humans to be vulnerable to fungus invasion. The rancid oils used in frying fast foods act as radical pollutants that get ingested and suppress immunity. Attacks on fungal organisms by a person's immune-system components would then lose much of their fungicidal effect. In addition, sugars, yeasts, and antibiotics in fast foods allow fungi to thrive.

SUPPLEMENTARY FACTORS FAVORING ATHLETE'S FOOT

Several factors increase your vulnerability to a fungus infection. First are the shoes you wear. In the modern closed shoe, the foot becomes hot and perspires. Excessive perspiration can cause maceration of the feet, which then feel soft and soggy, and can increase the alkalinity of the skin. The more alkaline the skin, the greater its receptivity to fungus.

Another factor is obesity. The added weight that the obese person carries might weaken the feet. Since weakened feet must constantly strain to accomplish their tasks, they perspire excessively and are then especially susceptible to infection.

FOOT FACT
During most of the 1980s, more than $2.7 billion per year was spent on athletic shoes in the United States.

By far, the Candida albicans, a one-celled fungus, is the most pervasive invader of the human body. Candida albicans derives from the phylum of plants with no chlorophyll and reproduces asexually by budding. Just one organism begets billions. It has a large, round, thick-walled spore shaped roughly like a tiny chicken egg. Upon entering a human, the organism seeks out the intestines, where its spores will dangle in clusters similar to bunches of grapes. The fungus then sends out its toxin to depress the immune system, allowing for fungal growth on other body parts. (In severe form, the organism can cause candidiasis, a systemic disease that requires treatment with immune-boosting ingredients.)

Impaired circulation also makes the feet receptive to an invasion of fungus. Furthermore, a debilitating disease such as arthritis or diabetes can stimulate the growth of fungi that have been lying dormant on the skin. Arthritis, especially rheumatoid arthritis and osteoarthritis, has been linked to athlete's foot. The perspiration of a diabetic is rich in sugar, making it a perfect medium for fungal bodies to thrive.

The final link in the chain of conditions that leads to athlete's foot is direct exposure to the fungus. If your feet are already susceptible when they come in contact with the fungus among us, infection might take place immediately. Such contact can be made through contaminated articles of clothing (shoes, slippers, stockings) or of personal use (towels, bathmats), or it can be made in public places where people walk barefoot. Whole families have become infected by the fungus as it spreads from one member to another. Epidemics have been common in schools, country clubs, and the armed forces. Entire armies of some small countries have been disabled by athlete's foot invasions.

WHO GETS ATHLETE'S FOOT?

Who gets athlete's foot? How old is he or she likely to be? Can it infect a person at any age? Has one's occupation anything to do with it?

Men are more commonly affected by athlete's foot than are women. The average American male is particularly susceptible because of the warmth, darkness, and moisture prevalent in his footgear. By preference or from occupational necessity, a man frequently wears heavy wool socks even on the warmest days. A heavy sock or even a light but nonabsorbent sock (one made of synthetic materials) worn inside a fully covered shoe on a hot day greatly increases the heat to which the foot is subjected. The foot perspires excessively, but the perspiration cannot be ventilated. Thus, the foot remains in a virtual steam bath the whole day long. The effect is to provide a hospitable atmosphere for the fungus that causes athlete's foot.

Women fare better than men because of the current trend in their shoe styles. Women's shoes are more open than men's and permit air and sunlight to reach the feet. Air evaporates the perspiration, and ultraviolet light from the sun helps control the fungus. Also, the sheerness of women's hosiery permits perspiration to evaporate more readily.

Persons between forty and fifty years of age are the ones most frequently subjected to athlete's foot. Their infections are recurrent, and the symptoms and signs—itching, scaling, and redness—are most evident during the summer months.

Next in order of frequency are people from ten to twenty years old. People that age are often active in school sports, dancing classes, and similar activities. The infections apparently result form direct barefoot contact with gymnasiums, locker rooms, shower rooms, or the area surrounding swimming pools.

Children ten or younger have a low incidence of infection. When children have their bathing, toenail clipping, and footgear selection supervised by parents, their feet do not afford the conditions that contribute to the infection. But after the age of six, children begin to bathe themselves and tend to their own personal hygiene, and they often do a poor job of it. The lack of proper parental supervision apparently opens the way for a primary invasion of tinea pedis.

Somewhat less affected by tinea pedis are adults from thirty to forty. Their cases often involve acute infections; they can experience itching, peeling, scaling, blisters, vesicles, pimples, fissures, burning, stinging, and more.

Adults from sixty to seventy display infections of a chronic type. Many of the cases in this group are men who were infected while serving in the armed forces during World War II or the Korean conflict. Their first symptoms might have been noticed as long as fifty years ago. Athlete's foot in this group can lie dormant for decades, then become active, occasionally leading to acute exacerbation, inflammation, and

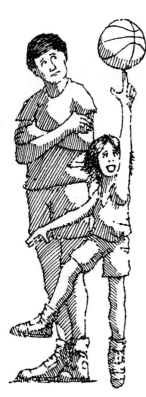

Men are more commonly affected by athlete's foot than are women.

blisters. More often than not, the toenails are involved and become a source of skin infection for other parts of the foot.

People over seventy who have athlete's foot display chronic fungus infections of the toenails. There are fewer patients in this group, but the affliction is prevalent, probably because elderly persons find it difficult to maintain good foot hygiene.

Occupation is definitely a factor in the incidence of athlete's foot. Bankers, brokers, and office workers who wear closed leather oxfords in summer and winter have tinea pedis more frequently than farmers, factory workers, and delivery persons. Because the worker at a sedentary occupation is often more subject to nervous tension and stress than is the manual worker, his perspiration is more likely to be alkaline – and an alkaline condition on the skin makes the feet susceptible to athlete's foot.

SYMPTOMS OF ATHLETE'S FOOT

Once a person has been affected by athlete's foot, whether fungus infection or allergic response to something in the environment, the symptoms appear quickly. More than one area of the foot is usually affected, but the problem, especially if it is from fungus, appears most often between the third and fourth toes and the fourth and fifth toes. Symptoms frequently develop in the longitudinal arches, in the toenails, and on the borders of the heel. The fungal invader can spread from the bottom of the foot to the top, and sometimes even to the hands.

The most frequent symptoms, in order of appearance, are scaling, itching, maceration, intertrigo, and tiny blisters.

Scaling, particularly between the toes, although not necessarily a sign of athlete's foot, is a prime cause for suspecting its presence. Scaling can be caused by athlete's foot, a circulatory disturbance, poor metabolism, nervousness, a vitamin deficiency, fatigue, or a systemic disease. The scale, which can be hard or soft, is a thin, plate-like structure. It is shed from the skin in pieces or in one large mass.

Itching is a symptom of athlete's foot, but it is not a specific indicator of a fungus infection. It can also be caused by an allergy, a skin eruption, a sunburn, or an overuse of drugs. It can be an outcome of swelling, nervousness, poor circulation, or a systemic disease such as diabetes or gout.

Maceration is a softening of the flesh. The skin wrinkles, frays, and peels. The condition is similar to the appearance of the feet after they have been in water a long time. Maceration is a symptom of athlete's foot, but it is also a primary symptom of intertrigo.

Intertrigo, which must be differentiated from a fungus infection, is sodden, moist, dead-appearing white skin surrounded by redness. It can be a direct result of rubbing an itch. Intertrigo must not be mistaken for athlete's foot. Treating it as such could cause an overtreatment burn from the application of excessively caustic medication.

Tiny blisters (vesicles) are the first *true* sign of a fungus infection. They might appear in groups and coalesce into large blisters, which then can break and expose the skin beneath. Those exposed areas are circular, shiny, red, and well defined. After a few days, the clear fluid in any blister that does not break is absorbed, leaving behind a brown spot. The roof of such a dry blister can tear and expose a red, smooth, shiny scale-covered surface.

If there is any change in circulation, or if the blisters break, there is a burning sensation. If the patient scratches the itch or rubs the burning area, then inflammation follows, creating heat, redness, and swelling. The swelling splits the skin, and fissures appear. After the blisters break, the skin peels and becomes inflexible and hard.

Finally, any motion of the foot causes pain. The skin surfaces rub against each other or against the inside of the shoe and are irritated. The pain may be eased by not moving the foot or by lubricating the skin around the toes.

The preceding symptoms are typical of the primary infection in athlete's foot. There can be a secondary infection, in which pus sacs form, and there can be blood poisoning. Should the infection be chronic, then hyperkeratosis—a thick, dry roughening of the skin—can also occur.

The pathogenic organisms that cause athlete's foot can thrive elsewhere in the body, too. They might also infect the head, the mouth, the inner thighs, the beard, the ears, the armpits, the trunk, and the hands. They are the same parasitical plant growths that cause other local manifestations, such as crumbling toenails and fingernails, jock itch, body rash, and more.

The fungus can also infect the toenails, which can reinfect the feet. This reinfection could become chronic. As the symptoms of athlete's foot appear, the patient usually tries to treat the infection himself. The symptoms diminish or disappear under the self-treatment but frequently reappear.

That analysis is corroborated by podiatrists everywhere around North America. The symptoms of athlete's foot recur in eighty percent of the cases from warm season to warm season; that is, for every five cases of athlete's foot, four are chronic. Although dryness and flaking might be more severe in winter because moisture evaporates from the skin in a heated room, the symptoms are generally less apparent during cold weather.

Podiatrists have reported at scientific meetings that they recognize a characteristic pattern in athlete's foot occurrences:

1. The patient acquires the condition in the spring or early summer.
2. The patient treats the athlete's foot himself or herself during the summer months.
3. The patient does not seek professional help until late September, after self-treatment probably has brought no improvement. By then, the self-treatment has caused either an allergic reaction to medications or associated complications on the hands.

That pattern of behavior is lamentable. For even if you do not realize you have athlete's foot, you cannot fail to recognize that your ailment deserves some medical attention. Self-treatment might certainly be successful; still, it tends to offer only a partial solution, for the disease usually recurs and must be treated professionally. If you suspect that your symptoms are caused by athlete's foot and self-treatment has failed you, then do not delay: go to your podiatrist or dermatologist at once.

FOOT FACT

Four out of five Americans own at least one pair of athletic shoes.

SELF-TREATMENT FOR ATHLETE'S FOOT

The symptoms of athlete's foot can be removed or reduced in ninety percent of the cases by following a procedure of excellent nutrition and topical application of remedies that have proven successful before. Here is what you can do for yourself:

1. Go to the health food store and purchase two bottles of Kyolic liquid. Kyolic is deodorized, aged, garlic extract that kills fungal organisms on contact.
2. In the morning, apply a thin coating of one bottle's worth of garlic liquid onto the feet, in particular where you have the fungal eruption. Cover the feet with plastic food wrap, pull on your hosiery, and go about your business for the day. You are forcing the aged garlic extract into the skin of your feet, where the fungal organisms are brought in close contact with an agent that kills them.
3. In the evening, soak your feet in a five percent solution of potassium permanganate contained in a gallon of purified water. You may acquire the little purple tablets of potassium permanganate as an over-the-counter remedy at your local drugstore. Soak your feet for at least an hour.
4. The following morning, open the second bottle of Kyolic. Make four garlic pills from the extract and the gelatin capsules that come in the Kyolic kit. Swallow the four garlic capsules with water. It's best to take two capsules following breakfast and two

following dinner. (For a more effective internal remedy, you can double the dose if garlic does not ordinarily upset your gastrointestinal system.) This internal remedy will be fungicidal in your gut the way it is on your feet. Unwelcome fungal overgrowth is probably involved with your intestinal digestive processes and potentially remains an ever-present source of reinfection.

To soothe feet made hot and inflamed by fungus or allergy, try dabbing plain, high-fat yogurt on the sore areas. Yogurt has friendly bacterial cultures as part of its nutritional ingredients, and certain of its bacteria kill off fungal organisms such as Candida albicans.

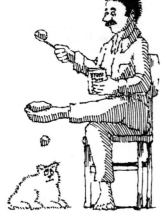

To soothe feet made hot and inflamed by fungus or allergy, try dabbing plain, high-fat yogurt on the sore areas.

Wearing open, ventilated shoes as much as possible might also help control the condition. A person who has athlete's foot should wear sandals or open-toe shoes. (In this case, it's the men who face the bigger challenge in bucking the fashion world and demanding to wear what they know is better for their feet.) Exposing the foot to air and sunlight is generally useful.

Your shoes deserve special attention because they are a major source of reinfection. Since the interior of shoes are never cleaned or washed, they often harbor the pathogenic fungi. For that reason alone, you should avoid wearing shoes without socks or stockings. Researchers could help the public greatly if they were to develop a good cleansing agent for footgear interiors. Such a cleanser would mechanically or chemically eliminate the debris that accumulates there—loose skin, dirt, thread, sweat, and other wastes.

Stockings and socks also become contaminated from contact with fungus. Ironing those articles can sterilize them; so can washing them in a medication that has been developed for that purpose.

HOW THE DOCTOR CAN HELP

Additionally, you can control athlete's foot by applying patent medicines recommended by your podiatrist. Anti-fungal powders, ointments, and liquids should be used as part of the morning routine when you are dressing for the day.

A podiatrist might give you griseofulvin, which is an anti-fungal antibiotic in pill form; he or she might give you copper sulphate electrical baths. Those procedures can effect a cure; in an all-out attack on fungus, they probably will be applied together. Many other professional athlete's foot remedies are available to your doctor, as well.

The treatment and ultimate control of athlete's foot is essential, but the primary goal is still the complete elimination of the condition. Podiatrists, family physicians, and dermatologists are striving toward that goal. However, nothing at present can take the place of preventive measures. If you wish to avoid the unpleasantness and discomfort of athlete's foot, you must practice good personal hygiene daily and care for your feet properly.

12. *Foot Odor*

ONE of the most annoying foot problems, although it is neither painful nor infectious, is known scientifically as bromidrosis; most of us would call it "smelly feet." You might rebel against the popular term, snicker at it, or consider the condition plainly distasteful to talk about, but the fact is that chronic foot odor afflicts several million Americans.

Marigold Susie Sambola, an instructor in weight control classes at the Young Women's Christian Association in Cleveland, has a heavy awareness of the evil smells emitted from some feet when folk remove their shoes and stand in their stockings or socks.

The obstacle to her breathing usually occurs between 5 and 7 p.m., when participants, mostly women, come to the YWCA's weight loss classes after having worked all day. During the course of receiving instruction, the people take off their shoes to be as light as possible for their weekly weigh-in.

When students step on the scale, the smell that wafts upward from their stockinged feet can be overwhelming, reports Marigold, who has to stand at the scale to record any weight change. "Not infrequently, I abruptly leave the room so as to gag in private and not embarrass my client. Often enough, that obese person has faced sufficient loss of confidence from being fat. In no way do I want to add to the individual's burden. So I breathe deeply outside the weigh-in room, then step back inside and resume my respirations with shallow breaths. Invariably, I must inhale through my mouth and try to hold my nostrils closed without putting fingers up to my nose."

The remedy for overcoming foot odor is not simple. Many people have a notion that bromidrosis is due only to a lack of cleanliness. "Why don't you wash your feet?" is often enough asked within the family circle when bromidrosis causes someone to rebel. There is a grain of truth to that, for proper foot hygiene will help. But foot odor is a genuine health problem that can be caused by factors other than a lack of washing. Those who suffer from the condition are subject to humiliating social situations such as the one occurring in Marigold Susie Sambola's weight control class.

Bromidrosis does not always yield quickly to treatment. It requires more than a washing of the feet to bring relief and eliminate the problem.

SYMPTOMS OF FOOT ODOR (IN ADDITION TO THE SMELL)

Bromidrosis, unpleasant and embarrassing for the victim, has a syndrome, or a group of signs and symptoms that accompany the smell. The entire smelly foot syndrome covers more than the obvious offense to one's nose. (Still, the nose knows!) The symptoms of bromidrosis are a sogginess of the skin between the toes and a tenderness of the flesh of the foot. In addition, there can be tiny blisters on the balls of the feet or on the heels.

Bromidrotic skin exhibits a weakness to infection, and fungus invasion is not uncommon. Indeed, athlete's foot and foot smell frequently go together. Their combination is a sign of general unhealthiness of the body or mind that sports them. We mention mind, because foot odor can indicate a certain perpetual mental tension of the sufferer—one of the four causes of this condition.

CAUSES OF BROMIDROSIS

The main cause of foot odor involves the presence of fetid bacteria on the foot, especially lodged between the toes. The fatty acids that are excreted in perspiration decompose in the presence of the fetid bacteria and generate an even fouler odor. This becomes especially noticeable in somebody who wears clothing derived from synthetic materials such as spandex, polyester, rayon, and nylon.

A functional disturbance in the nervous system—mental tension—is a second cause. Emotional stress stimulates body smell from tension sweat, which has its own distinct stink. A debilitating disease of the nerves or a blood dyscrasia such as anemia can lower one's resistance to disease and generate foot odor.

The ingestion of certain strong foods or spices, especially raw clove garlic, raw onions, freshly picked scallions, black pepper, and some others, can be a third cause of foot odor. The odoriferous products of those foods are predisposed to pass through the blood stream and eventually concentrate in the victim's perspiration.

The fourth, and perhaps most important, cause of foot odor is fatigue of the feet and legs. Foot fatigue, which might be related to one's occupation or to weak feet, will cause the lower limbs from the ankles down to perspire excessively.

Each cause relates directly or indirectly to perspiration. Foot and body perspiration, or generalized sweating, however, is not in itself a cause of bad odor. There is healthy perspiration caused by hard work or excessive heat, and there is unhealthy perspiration that derives from nervous tension. Healthy perspiration smells only when it is decomposed by fetid bacteria; unhealthy perspiration almost always has a distinctive odor. The stale odor of perspiration from nervous tension is often rather offensive.

A person who has bromidrosis is not always aware of his social handicap. But if he becomes self-conscious about it, he might suffer even more from nervous tension and thus produce more perspiration and more foot odor. This vicious cycle might induce the patient to visit a psychiatrist for treatment of the nervous condition rather than a podiatrist for treatment of the foot condition. If, however, the patient's nervous tension is not the cause of the foot odor, then the foot specialist or family doctor can help the odoriferous individual.

FOOT FACT

Each foot produces more than a cup of perspiration per day just in performing its job at the base of the body. When you exercise strenuously, each foot produces a lot more sweat—at least a pint.

TREATMENTS FOR FOOT ODOR

Washing the feet, changing the socks, and alternating the shoes every day are actions that anyone can take to help eliminate foot odor. They might not solve the problem, but they could help control it.

Professional care, however, often is needed to eliminate this vexing condition. A foot specialist can help in several ways. But he or she will be effective as a therapist only if the patient's problem has a local cause; that is, if it is traceable to the action of bacteria upon foot perspiration. Then, a variety of lotions, powders, and other remedies will be called upon for their therapeutic effects.

A consulting podiatrist is likely also to check the diet to ascertain whether the patient has been eating spices or other strong-odored foods. If the patient has been consuming foodstuffs that might contribute to the smell, he or she will be advised to eliminate them from the diet. If the podiatrist suspects that a constitutional disease might be causing the bromidrosis, he or she will, of course, refer the patient to a physician for a thorough physical examination.

Once a foot doctor has determined that the cause of the foot odor is local, he or she will recommend any or all of several methods of treatment.

First, of course, the foot specialist probably will advise the patient to bathe the feet with warm water and soap at least once a day. He or she might also suggest changing to white cotton socks in summer or to lightweight woolen hose in winter. The doctor will also insist that shoes be aired thoroughly for at least twenty-four hours after wearing. The patient must alternate pairs of shoes, never wearing the same pair two days in a row.

After establishing the rules to follow for good foot hygiene, the podiatrist most likely will use special methods to treat the foot odor. One of the health professional's best procedures is to administer a zinc sulphate medicinal electrical bath, which reduces the perspiration. The bath tends to shrink the sweat glands so that they excrete less moisture that can be decomposed by the fetid bacteria. An average of two such baths a week for several weeks often helps.

In conjunction with the bath, a foot doctor may use various modalities to keep the feet dry. A five percent solution of formalin in alcohol is effective when applied daily as a lotion. (Perhaps two or three times a week is sufficient, too.) A solution of one part of potassium permanganate to a thousand parts of water applied once a day for ten minutes is known to give good results. It does stain clothing, however, and probably should be applied when the patient can allow the feet enough time to dry.

Upon arising, the patient should sprinkle into his or her shoes a good dry foot powder. The powder will absorb the moisture that accumulates inside the footgear and in the fibers of absorbent socks.

Germicidal agents can be useful when put directly on the feet to destroy the local bacteria. Even underarm deodorants might be helpful for that purpose

HOMEOPATHIC REMEDIES

Homeopathy is a scientific method of stimulating the body's own healing processes to cure illnesses. It is a system of medical treatment based on the use of minute quantities of a substance to cure the effects that are produced by larger quantities of that very same substance. (Homeopathy gets its name from the Greeks; *homoios* means similar, and *pathos* means suffering.)

William J. Faber, doctor of osteopathy and medical director of the Milwaukee Pain Clinic, uses some highly effective homeopathic remedies to overcome all forms of hyperhidrosis (excessive sweating), including the kind that leads to the fetid sweat odor of smelly feet. Dr. Faber treats numerous patients who are in a state of high tension resulting from pain. Such tension brings on tension sweating, often associated with foot and body odor. Dr. Faber recommends that such a foot odor victim apply a topical homeopathic product called BHI Perspiration. Specifically recommended for offensive foot sweat, it is patted on the skin of the lower limbs and offers no side effects. (The product contains jaborandi, saliva officinalis, sambucus nigra, cedron, acidum nitricum, petroleum, sanguinaria canadensis, thuja occidentalis, acidum salicylicum, acidum sulphuricum, calcarea carbonica, and sepia. It is produced for doctors by Biologic Homeopathic Industries, in Albuquerque, New Mexico. For further information, call the company at [800] 621-7644 or [505] 293-3843.)

If neither homeopathic nor more conventional applications overcome your bromidrosis, then ask your physician, podiatrist, or chiropractor to supply you with either adrenal substance or hypothalamus—glandular homeopathic remedies that can be taken internally. Those glandulars are food supplements, not drugs, and therefore might also be available in health food stores.

Most allopathic physicians use drug therapies, which work opposite to the way homeopathic remedies act; consequently, the traditionally trained physician is likely to resist the use of homeopathic treatments. You'll probably have to try those remedies on your own.

OVERCOMING EMBARRASSMENT

Whether a manifestation of inner turmoil or of poor foot hygiene, bromidrosis is always a source of embarrassment. It will not disappear by itself, and it cannot be wished away. One has to make a genuine effort to eliminate it. The podiatrist might not be able to help if the problem is caused by nervous tension—that could be a task for a psychiatrist. But a foot specialist can combat foot odor that is caused by the combination of bacteria and excessive perspiration.

You don't have to be embarrassed by smelly feet.

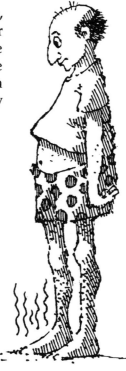

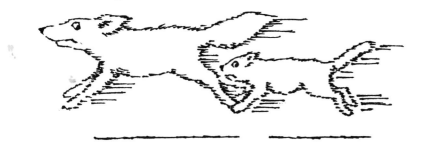

13. *Metatarsalgia: A Nerve Pain*

ONE-THIRD of all women who live in industrialized western countries and frequently dress fashionably will, at some time in their lives, be struck by a sudden, sharp, stabbing pain in the toes of one or both feet. The pain might come and go intermittently. It could linger for years, coming on sporadically for no apparent reason, then go away forever. Or, it can remain a prolonged and continuous agony and then disappear—returning again when least expected and, of course, never wanted. It might hit during a trek in the woods or while shopping in the supermarket. It can come over the toes to produce a spasm of pain and leave just as suddenly. It may strike the toes of men, as well, but seldom with the violent distress with which it strikes the toes of women.

The victim's condition, metatarsalgia (sometimes called Morton's toe), is not, however, derived from the individual's toes. Instead, it's a neuralgia, an inflammation of the nerve between the third and fourth metatarsal bones. (See Figure 13.1.)

CAUSES OF METATARSALGIA

Metatarsalgia comes about by the compression of a small toe nerve between two displaced metatarsal bones. Inflammation occurs when the head of one displaced metatarsal presses against another and catches the nerve between them. With every step, the nerve is pushed together by the bones and then rubbed, pressed again, and irritated

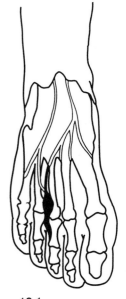

Figure 13.1
Metatarsalgia gives the toes agonizing pain. It is caused by an inflammation of the nerve between the third and fourth metatarsal bones. The shaded area shows the nerve thickening and a tumor forming.

without relief. Consequently, the surrounding nerve tissue becomes enlarged with a sheath of scar tissue that forms to protect the nerve fibers.

If you suspect that the shoe plays a role in this ailment, as it does in many other foot problems, then you have reasoned correctly. But it's not just any type of shoe. Women are the chief victims of this toe pain; they experience metatarsalgia as a result of wearing high-style shoes that sport fashionably elevated heels and pointed toes. Metatarsalgia can affect men, as well, if they constantly wear tight shoes or the pointed-toe Italian styles that compress their feet in a similar way to those fashionable women's shoes.

Shoes that are too tight actually force the metatarsal bones to drop at their heads. The metatarsals become displaced. The foot becomes malformed. Here's how:

The anterior metatarsal arch runs across the foot where the toes join the metatarsals. (See Figure 1.2.) It is slight, but it normally flexes up and down in walking as weight is placed on the foot and then removed. As this arch flexes, the foot becomes somewhat broader. Yet, if the ends of the arch are rigidly fixed by shoes that are too tight, then there is no room for the arch to move. The weight of walking can then force one of the metatarsals out of place. It drops. All the metatarsals can fall. The anterior arch might be eliminated completely. In fact, where the bottom of the foot was once concave, the dropped metatarsals might make it convex.

Women's shoes in particular will cause metatarsalgia. A high-heeled shoe puts undue stress and strain on the front of the foot by sliding it forward and downward on the curved shank of the shoe. The tapered-toe style adds to the pressures on the metatarsals by squeezing the bones together until they strike the intervening nerve, creating friction. Both of those shoe styles—overly high heels and needle-nose toes—contribute to the causes of metatarsalgia.

SELF-HELP CARE FOR METATARSALGIA

You can temporarily relieve the sudden sharp stab of pain that signals metatarsalgia by using simple common-sense measures and some home remedies.

Imagine you are dressed in an evening gown and attending the President's ball. It's an evening involving much dancing in your high-fashion slippers. When not foxtrotting around the room, you are standing on unyielding marble floors and performing the rituals of cocktail sipping, introducing friends, being introduced by them, shouting inconsequential small talk amid the din of dozens of people, and generally observing others as you are being observed yourself. Standing in the vise-like grip of torturous footgear that looks so pretty but makes you feel as if hot pokers are coursing along your foot tissues, you are longing to sit down. And then the pain that you've learned to dread arrives. You ache! It's like an arrow has been shot into your third and fourth toes. What do you do?

Sit down, of course. Remove your shoe and massage the foot. Bend the toes and elongate them. Massage between the metatarsal bones, as well as the area where the pain seems to be located. Put your thumb under the ball of your foot; with your other fingers, grasp the toes. Press upward with the thumb while pushing downward and forward with the other fingers. That should stretch the nerves into the toes, thus interrupting the pain cycle and providing immediate relief. Perform as needed.

Moreover, cold sensations often provide temporary relief. Try stepping barefoot on a cold floor (marble is marvelous). You might try holding a wrapped ice cube against the painful area to cool the nerve and take away the heat of inflammation. With nerve pains, there's no telling what will give comfort.

A more permanent way to give yourself relief is to remove pressure from the affected nerve orthopedically. The burning, cramping pain might be countered by placing a felt pad just under the ball of the foot. Put such a pad inside your shoe under the sock lining. When placed just right, the pad removes pressure from the nerve sheath (which by now has been enlarged by fluid accumulation and possibly has become an actual tumor). Thus, the irritation will cease somewhat.

You can also help yourself through stretching exercises (see chapter twenty) or by wearing low-heel shoes. Slashing open the shoes will give your tortured toes more room in which to spread out. If you find that none of those methods relieves the acute pain of metatarsalgia, then you should seek surgical care from a podiatrist.

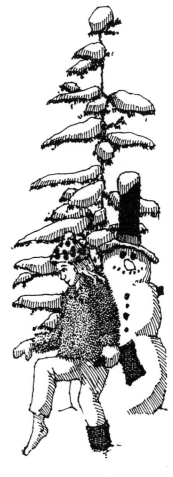

Cold sensations often
provide temporary relief.

PROFESSIONAL CARE FOR METATARSALGIA

When relief from metatarsalgia is needed, a foot specialist works more dramatically and more swiftly than the usual self-help methods. Let's face it—the podiatrist is trained and has the medicines and instruments for providing such comfort. Injection of a local anesthetic into the foot will relieve symptoms immediately and reduce the inflammation by stimulating blood circulation in the area. The podiatrist gives the injection and repeats it daily until the pain disappears.

If the irritation has been present a long time, scar tissue around the nerve can develop into a tumor. It's standard operating technique for podiatric surgeons to remove that tumor surgically. Their office procedures employ the modern way of doing things. Avoid hospitalization, if you can.

Before surgery is attempted, every other available method of relief is usually tried. For instance, placing a transverse bar across the outside of the shoe sole, elevating the foot, and applying warm moist packs can all give relief. A more efficient type of help is available through an orthotic appliance that relieves the strain on the affected long bones in the foot. It works better than self-administered padding of the shoes. The orthotic fits your arch and elevates the heads of the metatarsal bones. Because the appliance is removable, it can be worn in almost any pair of shoes.

Still, nothing might help much when it comes to a nerve pain such as metatarsalgia. Self-care and podiatric care via padding, injections, physical therapy, and other ministrations might need improving upon. That's when surgical removal of the tumor might have to be instituted.

IN-OFFICE SURGERY

Dedicated marathon runner Freida K., age 30, sought relief from the regularly occurring pain she felt in the space between the third and fourth toes of her right foot. The condition was diagnosed as Morton's toe. Palliative treatment was administered through injection therapy and then orthopedics, but nothing brought permanent relief. The pain would leave Freida's foot for up to a week but always returned. Finally, the doctor recommended surgery to remove the tumor that had grown between the woman's metatarsal bones.

Freida carefully considered her situation. The metatarsalgia was causing her much discomfort. Worse for her, she was unable to feel secure during her running, and that brought about several race defeats when ordinarily she would have won. So she decided to have the operation.

Indeed, it was an easy surgery, undergone right there in the doctor's office. She found it unnecessary to take any painkillers, because discomfort during convalescence was tolerable. She remained completely ambulatory and did not lose any time from work. Six weeks after the procedure, she began practicing for her next marathon. Freida K. said, "This is the easiest operation anyone could undergo. I think it's the greatest. And my health insurance paid for the whole thing."

FOOT FACT

The biggest boost athletic shoes ever got was from the prolonged New York City transit strike in 1980. That's when trendy—and sensible—people started wearing running shoes and tennis sneakers to walk to work, and they have not given them up since.

14. *Heel Spurs: A Toothache in Your Foot*

THE problems podiatrists see most frequently—corns, calluses, bunions, metatarsalgia, and other common troubles—usually involve the toes. But heel spurs, which come from an anatomical change of the calcaneus (heel bone), involve one's heel area and occasionally some type of systemic disability such as arthritis.

The heel spur, or calcaneal spur, is a nail-like growth of calcium around the ligaments and tendons of the foot where they attach to the heel bone. The spur grows from the bone and into the flesh of the foot. It might take years to become a problem, but once it appears, it will cause considerable suffering.

Because of its proximity to tendons, the spur is a source of continuous painful aching. The sensation is like a toothache is in your foot. In fact, on X-ray examination, the spur can resemble a protruding tooth penetrating the flesh of the heel.

When you place your weight on the heel, the pain can be sufficient to immobilize you. Anyone—athlete, office worker, outdoor laborer, housewife, or weightlifter—can be affected. Women and men are equally apt to suffer from it.

Age and health have something to do with its occurrence. The calcaneal spur is seen most often in persons who are past forty. The condition might also be associated with osteoarthritis, rheumatoid arthritis, poor circulation of the blood, and other degenerative diseases.

THE CAUSE OF HEEL SPURS

To understand why and how the spur may appear, one must understand the architecture and operation of the foot. The heel bone forms one end of the two longitudinal arches of the foot. (See Figures 1.3 and 1.4.) Those arches are held together by ligaments and are activated by the muscles of the foot, some of which are attached beneath the arches and run from the front of the foot to the back. Those muscles and ligaments, like the other supporting tissues of the body, are attached in two places. Many are attached at the heel bone.

The strain upon those muscles as they perform their tasks is the cause of the calcaneal spur. The body reacts to the stress at the heel bone by calcifying the soft tissue attachments. They get hard as stone at the attachment places, and this hardening produces the spurring effect that hurts so much. You really could say that you have a tooth growing in your heel and that it needs pulling.

The strain that produces the spur can be caused by weak feet, prolonged standing, or improper shoes. In each case, the feet are inadequate for the tasks they must perform. For spurs to form, the strain must be continuous; it might take many years for an overgrowth of calcification to develop.

SYMPTOMS OF CALCANEAL SPURRING

The pain caused by a calcaneal spur is not the result of the pressure of weight on the point of the spur, but of inflammation around the tendons where they attach to the heel bone. You might expect the pain to increase as you walk on the spur, but actually it decreases. The pain is most severe when you start to walk after a rest.

What happens is that the nerves and capillaries adapt themselves to the situation as you walk; when you rest, the nerves and capillaries also rest. Then, as you begin to move about again, extreme demands are made on the blood vessels. The rush of blood to the inflamed area around the calcaneal spur shocks those nerves and capillaries into pain, which continues until they again adjust to the spur. If excessive strain had been placed on the foot the day before, the pain might now be very great. A sudden strain, such as might be produced by leaping or jumping, can also increase the pain.

The pain might be localized at first. There will seem to be one central spot that is the root of the trouble, but continued walking and standing will soon cause the entire heel to become tender and painful. The hurt is rather distinctive.

The spur can cause a change in the normal gait. In an effort to protect the heel and minimize the pain, the sufferer might favor one

FOOT FACT

The most common foot injury is plantar fasciitis (also known as strained plantar fascia), which is a pain under and in front of the heel.

foot. Soon, excessive use of the non-painful foot will likely lead to both feet being affected. If there are spurs in both heels, one could be more painful than the other. Favoring the more painful foot will simply accelerate the growth of the spur in the other. Both feet will then give acute discomfort.

HOME-CARE RELIEF FOR HEEL SPURS

You can try to get relief from a painful heel spur by treatment at home. Obviously, you should rest the foot as much as possible. Elevate the foot to reduce pressure upon the inflamed area. Apply heat to the painful area. The heat will ease the pain by dilating your local blood vessels. Dilation allows the blood to circulate more freely so as to carry away fluids that cause swelling—and it's the swelling that causes the pain.

One can also protect the heel by placing a foam rubber pad in the heel of the shoe. A pad about a half-inch thick will raise the heel, shift the weight of the body forward, and protect the irritated muscles attached to the heel bone.

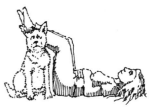

Elevate the foot to reduce pressure upon the inflamed area.

The same effect can be achieved by using adhesive tape to turn the foot inward. Apply one-inch-wide by one-foot-long strips to the bottom of the foot, directly in front of the painful area, and then pull upward and make snug to the ankle. This treatment will relax the short foot muscles and take the strain off the heel bone. One can also accomplish the same effect by having a shoemaker place an inner-sole wedge or a transverse bar on the shoe sole. Those treatments will eliminate the symptoms in a few weeks—if the condition has not been present long enough to establish a pain syndrome.

HOW FOOT SPECIALISTS TREAT HEEL SPURS

If none of the methods of self-treatment gives relief, then you most likely will need to go to a podiatrist for permanent relief. He or she has many methods for correcting the pain of heel spurs. Some involve surgery, but others do not.

After the foot specialist has diagnosed the problem to his satisfaction and has taken and analyzed X-ray films of the inflamed area, he might treat the spur with any number of physical therapies, such as diathermy, ultrasound waves, and whirlpool baths. The diathermy treatment uses an electric current to produce heat that sedates the inflamed tissues. The ultrasound device sends sound waves into the heel and sets up a massaging action that stimulates blood circulation. Treatment with a whirlpool bath involves placing the foot directly into the jetting stream; again, a gentle massaging action is induced.

Orthopedic molds and appliances, such as orthotics, are designed by foot specialists for use inside the shoe to eliminate irritation to the heel when the patient stands or walks. A horseshoe- or doughnut-shaped pad can be applied to relieve the pressure at the point of pain and to redistribute over a wider area the weight that ordinarily lies on the heel. When those appliances are used, the spur, in effect, floats in air. At the same time, the body's weight is transferred forward from the tender spot.

Heel spurs are extremely painful. Furthermore, no non-surgical treatment can give immediate relief from the pain. Surgery, which is a more radical treatment, has proven itself as a permanent correction. You and the doctor might consider it a last resort when relief and cure can be obtained no other way, but heel surgery does rid you of the spur. If the podiatrist believes that surgery is indicated, he will recommend an operation—but only after establishing that less-drastic methods of treatment are not going to do the job.

SURGICAL CORRECTION OF HEEL SPURS

"The removal of a painful spur from the heel of Joe DiMaggio is what cut short his baseball career," said Dr. Albert Brown, a retired ambulatory foot surgeon. "The orthopedic surgeon who excised the large bony prominence from DiMaggio's heel bone produced a surgical scar almost six inches long. It took thirty stitches to close."

That kind of extensive procedure does not have to be performed anymore. The operation isn't even done in the hospital; rather, the whole thing takes place in the foot doctor's office.

Back in 1962, a clinical journal published an article by Dr. Brown describing for the first time his technique for removal of such a heel spur—a procedure performed without pain, under local anesthesia, and without the need for the hospitalization that Joe DiMaggio required.

Lorraine O. was severely troubled by a chronically painful ache in her heel. She sought relief for her heel spur from a foot doctor who first employed the conservative therapy of strapping and padding the heel. But long-lasting relief eluded the patient no matter how much physical therapy and how many painkillers were tried. Consequently, the doctor recommended heel surgery as a last resort. He did the operation in his office.

Ambulatory foot surgeons characteristically attempt milder methods before suggesting operative procedures. But in Lorraine's case, the milder treatment was not sufficient to cope with the gigantic size of her calcaneal spur.

Instead, Lorraine's entire heel spur was removed—but through a mere quarter-inch incision on the inner side of the heel. She wore regular shoes throughout the healing period. She was hardly distracted from her everyday tasks after the operation, and she continued to work as a cashier in a busy restaurant. She said, "I am so happy to be rid of this toothache in my foot."

15. *Weak Arches and Flat Feet*

THE thought of other individuals' having flat feet is humorous to some unaffected people. But there is nothing funny in it for anyone who suffers from weak arches and flat feet. The two conditions, so uniquely human, practically always go together.

Policemen who walk a beat have earned the nickname "flatfoot," but they are not the only ones who traditionally have fallen arches; so do letter carriers, waiters, dentists, meter maids, house painters, and many others who walk or stand on their feet for hours. Even people who never spend much time on their feet can have fallen arches.

Flat feet are not entirely beyond remedy. That's because, first of all, flat feet are usually not completely flat (although they might eventually become so if the condition is not corrected early on). Thus, many foot specialists maintain that the description "fallen arches" is misleading and that the condition should properly be called "weak arches." To the sufferer, "fallen arches" is descriptive enough. (The two terms are used interchangeably in this book.)

ANATOMICAL BREAKDOWN OF "FALLEN ARCHES"

In the classic instance of so-called fallen arches, nearly all the bones of the foot change position. The heel bone rolls inward, the ankle drops, the shin becomes more prominent, the cuboid bone forces outward, and both the big toe and the fifth toe rise. The other bones sink, and the inner longitudinal arch "falls." The anatomical breakdown resulting from fallen arches is classical and distinctive.

If, at any point, you suspect that pains in your legs or feet might be coming from fallen arches, you can initially check it yourself. The surest sign of weak feet with arches ready to fall is an actual flatness of the feet. If you observe that they are flat as pancakes, then you probably do have fallen arches. Another test is to stand before a mirror and try to observe the backs of your bare feet. Notice whether the heel tendons bow inward, like a pair of inverted parentheses. If you then stand on the outer margins of your feet and the tendons straighten out, you probably have fallen arches.

A foot doctor, of course, can verify those suspicions with an X-ray photograph, which would clearly show any alteration in the position of the bones.

SYMPTOMS OF WEAK ARCHES

The symptoms that accompany weak arches are a feeling of pain and burning in the foot and a tiredness and aching pain in the legs, especially after standing or walking. Painful calluses grow on the ball of the foot because the anterior metatarsal arch also falls.

The effects of fallen arches vary from victim to victim. The amount of pain in each case is determined by the severity of the individual anatomical breakdown.

The most troublesome symptom is the painful feeling in the feet and legs. In addition, fatigue is always present, not only in the lower extremities but in the back. Back pain is often evident, because the muscles in the back tense and strain as they try to compensate for the weak muscles and the structural imbalance in the feet.

The legs might swell or be puffy above the ankle. Sometimes, the weakened feet have a purplish discoloration. Also, there is pain and tenderness when the center of the soles are pressed.

The toes can deform. Other difficulties, such as bunions, bursitis, and calluses, might develop. If lower limb circulation is poor, then fallen arches can also produce a sensation of heaviness and congestion, as if heavy bricks were inside the shoes.

When arches fall, the foot increases in both length and width, making it more difficult to buy footgear that fits properly.

Why do those symptoms occur? Why, in fact, do arches "fall" in the first place?

Weak arches with flattening of the feet result from the inability of the feet to bear the body's weight. The body, in effect, demands more of the feet than they can perform. Those demands are prolonged; the strain upon the feet is there day after day after day. Sooner or later, if no relief is given, the arches weaken and fall.

WHY ARCHES FALL

Whether we call the condition fallen arches, weak arches, or flat feet, its mechanics are simply explained. The bones of each foot form a complex structure of four arches. Displacement of any one bone will weaken the position of another by placing additional strain upon the ligaments and muscles that help hold that other bone in place. The effect can be visualized by imagining an arch of wooden blocks held together by a network of elastic bands. Continued pressure at the top of the arch might not cause the whole structure to fall immediately, but it can force one of the blocks out of place. Once that has happened, and given time and sufficient pressure at the top of the arch, all the blocks will give way eventually. That is what happens when the arches of your feet fall.

That example illustrates two conditions that contribute to fallen arches: time and weight. The most obvious source of fallen arches is excess body weight. An increase in the size of the load that your feet have to carry places them under a greater strain. Excessive weight causes the feet to weaken. The ligaments and muscles stretch or tear, and the bones of the foot drop. Therefore, obesity can cause fallen arches.

The case histories of flatfooted victims such as waitresses, postal clerks, salespeople, schoolteachers, homemakers, department store floor walkers, and nurses—all of whom must frequently stand or walk for long hours while they work—prove that prolonged foot strain produces weak arches. The muscles of the feet would then be less prepared for the additional demands placed upon them after age forty, when there is a tendency to exercise less and to overeat. The increased weight, the weakened muscles, and the long hours of strain lead to chronic foot fatigue, which, in turn, can lead to fallen arches.

Other factors that can lead to weak arches are rickets, sudden injury, malnutrition, infection, and, possibly, inappropriate footgear (such as wearing sandals for hiking on mountain trails). The arches of congenitally weak feet—those that do not have muscles and ligaments of sufficient strength to bear the body's normal weight—might fall, but in such instances there is no special cause except, perhaps, heredity.

Generally, shoes contribute to fallen arches in women only. Because the high-heeled, pointed-toe shoe is not really suitable for standing and walking, it contributes to foot strain and general fatigue. Consequently, more women than men have flat feet.

Fallen arches can lead to arthritis of the foot, for the pressures on the foot that ultimately cause the arches to weaken might also inflame and irritate the ligaments that hold the bones in place. The body reacts to the irritation and inflammation by protecting the surface of the joints with fluid. As the body continues to produce fluid, the pressure on the joints increases. They become further inflamed, and arthritis results.

FOOT FACT

Flat feet and feet with very high arches usually function quite well without correction.

HOME-CARE RELIEF—BUT NOT A CURE—FOR FLAT FEET

Adults who have flat feet cannot be cured. The feet will remain flat. Relief is all that any treatment can achieve, although long-lasting relief might be obtained by supporting and protecting the arch with flexible foot molds. Devices that support the arch have been used for years, but rigid arch supports are used most often by children. If the mold or arch support is properly made over a plaster or plastic replica of the foot or on the foot itself, it will reduce the strain immediately.

When the pain from fallen arches is sudden and acute, you can obtain some relief at home by elevating and resting the foot and by applying hot packs. Moist warm towels placed over the foot and leg will give some relief, as will infrared radiation from a heat lamp. As the inflammation diminishes, a gentle massaging of the foot muscles will be soothing.

TREATMENT BY FOOT SPECIALISTS

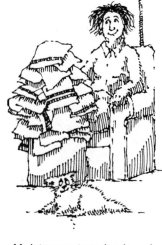

Moist warm towels placed over the foot and leg will give some relief.

A foot specialist can help you by using adhesive tape to support the arches. First, the doctor applies two strips of inch-wide adhesive around the borders of the sole of the foot. The strips run back from the fifth metatarsal head, along the outer side of the foot, around the heel, and forward along the inner side of the foot to the first metatarsal head. Then he places five long strips of adhesive tape, in an overlapping manner, down the leg and under the arch. Each strip runs diagonally from the outer side of the middle third of the leg, across the shin and the inner side of the foot, under the arch, then up across the shin and back again to the middle third of the leg, this time on the inner side.

This strapping, known as an X strap because the strips of tape cross at the shin, supports the arch and anchors the heel. The two strips push the heel upward and inward; the five long strips raise and support the longitudinal arches. On about the fourth day, the strapping will start to fray at the edges; it therefore will need to be changed after four to six days. The taping continues until all discomfort from fallen arches stays away permanently. The strapping can be worn when bathing.

Felt pads can give similar support to the arches. Either place the pads in the shoes or tape them beneath the arches of the feet.

Perhaps the best therapy for acutely flat feet is a warm whirlpool bath. The bath, which requires a stainless steel tub that holds twenty or more gallons of water, is valuable in precisely such circumstances. An electric motor jets a stream of air into the warm water and causes it to revolve turbulently. The effect when the podiatrist places your feet in the water is a gentle buffeting that sets up a massaging action. The water massage penetrates deep into the feet and stimulates circulation in the inflamed and painful muscles, ligaments, and joints. A whirlpool bath may, of course, be used to treat other foot ailments; it is particularly effective at relieving the pain of inflammation. When it eliminates the inflammation, the pain goes away. It should not be used, however, if a patient is suffering from phlebitis (inflammation of a vein).

The foot doctor can also employ other methods of physical therapy. One for which there is no substitute is the use of the doctor's own skilled hands to provide relief by manipulating the bones and muscles of the foot. The doctor may also use ultrasound waves, heat lamps, diathermy, galvanism, and paraffin baths.

Providing relief from pain is one goal in the treatment of flat feet, but correction of the deformity is even more important. Correction, in the sense of restoring normal or near-normal functioning to the damaged muscles and ligaments, is possible in many cases. Unfortunately, it is not possible in all cases.

The relief gained from taping the arches, from resting the foot, and from applying heat and massage, whether at home or by means of the podiatrist's physical therapy, is temporary. If nothing is done to address the fallen arches, then there will be periodic episodes of pain as the symptoms appear, are treated, disappear, then appear again. The podiatrist can halt that cycle. Once the foot doctor has succeeded in removing the inflammation and the initial symptoms, he or she can devise appliances to prevent recurrence. Those appliances, whether of plastic, metal, leather, cork, rubber, or felt, support and protect the irritated muscles and joints. They are fitted to the foot as false teeth are fitted to the gums. The podiatrist makes or builds the appliances to conform exactly to the needs of the fallen arches.

EXTERNAL CORRECTIONS APPLIED TO SHOES

Corrective devices can also be placed on the sole of the shoe. The Thomas heel, the comma-shaped bar, and the transverse bar have been used to correct the bone displacement that occurs in weak feet with fallen arches. (See Figure 15.1.) Those shoe devices are sometimes effective even when all other means of correction have failed.

The Thomas heel is a specially shaped heel that is half an inch longer than a normal heel; it projects forward on the inside of the foot to a point near the center of the inner longitudinal arch. It is also slightly (1/16 to 1/8 inch) higher on the inside than on the outside. Its wedge shape changes the balance of the heel and exerts a twisting force on the bones of the arches. The effect, similar to stepping on a nickel with the inner edge of the heel, is sufficient to cause the toes to turn inward to a pigeon-toed position.

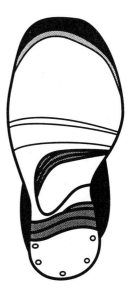

Figure 15.1
Shoe corrections such as (from bottom to top) the Thomas heel, the comma-shaped bar, and the transverse bar often work together to relieve the strain of weak foot muscles.

Both the transverse bar, placed near the front of the shoe sole to support the metatarsals, and the comma-shaped bar, placed near the middle of the sole to support the arches, can be used in conjunction with the Thomas heel. Although the bars differ in shape and give support to different areas of the sole of the foot, they both elevate the anterior metatarsal arch and alter the position of the bones of the foot.

The comma-shaped bar is 1/8-inch higher at the "tail" on the outer side of the shoe sole (behind the fifth metatarsal head) than at the "dot" on the inner side. That elevation causes the front of the foot to twist outward. With a Thomas heel raising the inner side of the heel and the comma-shaped bar raising the outer side of the ball of the foot, the longitudinal arches are twisted. In consequence, circulation increases, and muscle structure is toned.

Anyone with flat feet and weak arches would be well advised to seek help. Podiatrists have specialized in diagnosing and treating countless foot problems. From an examination of the feet and of X-ray photographs, they can determine which structures are at fault and which need correction. Because podiatrists are well qualified to construct devices and supports that will meet the specific problem, they can provide sufferers long-lasting relief from the pain of fallen arches.

16. *Sudden Injury: Ankle Sprains*

CORNS and bunions develop slowly. So do many other foot ailments that are caused by continued abuse of the feet—perhaps by improper attention to foot care. Indeed, most foot troubles develop so slowly that you could be but vaguely aware of discomfort. Ultimately, of course, you will have to deal with the problem through a program of self-help or by bringing your difficulties to a foot specialist. But the initial discomfort from a common foot ailment might not goad you to seek medical attention at once.

Sprained ankles are different from other foot problems, since they occur in an instant. The moment you sprain an ankle, you are aware of it; the injury is sudden, the damage immediate. Moreover, you will want, and need, professional medical attention. That much should be obvious to anyone who has ever sprained an ankle.

An ankle sprain, common among those who have weak feet, wear high heels, or use shoes with run-down heels, is a result of a violent twisting of the foot. You may sprain an ankle quite casually as you stroll along the street. You might experience a sprain when you step upon an uneven surface, such as a rock or a curbstone; when you catch the toe of your shoe in a grating; or when you jump from any height. The more active you are, the greater the possibility that you will undergo an ankle sprain. Sprains, of course, are not always the result of strenuous activity, but they can be expected by anyone who does much running, jumping, or leaping. Sprains of the ankles are, in fact, quite common among athletes in many sports.

SIGNS AND SYMPTOMS OF ANKLE SPRAIN

Since a sprain occurs when the foot is twisted, it is most likely to happen when the foot is somehow off-balance. When the weight of the body comes down on only one side of the foot, it is not transmitted directly to the ground. When the foot is off-balance and the body's weight is suddenly thrust upon it, the strain is greater than the ligaments can withstand. Consequently, the ligaments that connect the anklebone to the shinbone tear. The more violently the ankle is twisted, the greater the damage and pain.

Immediately after the sprain, the signs and symptoms of injury appear. Placing any weight directly on the injured foot can cause pain. If the sprain is slight, the ankle becomes tender and sensitive. If the sprain is severe, the ankle might become hot, swollen, tender, and so painful that you cannot walk. The ankle becomes discolored, sometimes red, sometimes blue. As the swelling increases, it is accompanied by throbbing.

In a severe sprain of the ankle, a bone fragment might be pulled loose from the shinbone where the torn ligament had been attached. Therefore, every sprain of this part of the anatomy should be X-rayed. Possible fractures can be diagnosed only by examination of the X-ray photographs.

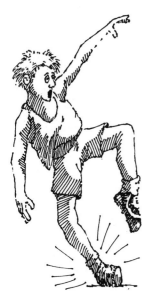

EMERGENCY SELF-TREATMENT FOR ANKLE SPRAIN

Suppose you're playing basketball and that after taking a layup you come down hard on an awkwardly bent ankle. You sustain a bad sprain that forces you to leave the game. If there is no medical attention available at the site, then what's to be done on an emergency basis for self-treatment?

Treatment of a sprained ankle should begin even before you get to a doctor. First, take your weight off the ankle. Sit down. After such injury you must not use the foot. The seriousness of the injury cannot always be determined immediately, for the symptoms don't appear all at once. The sprain might seem to be only a temporary impediment, but using the ankle can easily increase the damage. Don't take the risk. When a sprain is truly severe, this warning is scarcely necessary, because in such cases walking will cause considerable pain.

The next step is to reduce the swelling and throbbing. Apply cold wet cloths or ice packs to the ankle at once. After a lapse of time, warm applications, which will increase the circulation to the area and diffuse the swelling, might be of more value.

Once those steps have reduced the swelling and throbbing, you must devise a proper support for the ankle until you can see a foot doctor. Bandage the sprain by wrapping a roll of three-inch gauze around the ankle from the toes to just below the knee. To prevent ankle motion from side to side, tape two-foot-long strips of inch-wide adhesive around the gauze to secure it in place. The ankle support that you want to produce should permit heel-to-toe movement while bracing the ankle against side-to-side motion. Since heel-to-toe movement is usually painless, the foot can be used for walking straight forward once the swelling has been reduced somewhat and the ankle has been supported with gauze and tape. You can give the injured part additional support by placing the foot in a high shoe or a high-top sneaker snugly laced.

Those emergency steps will suffice until you get to a foot specialist. Go to one. Even if the pain and discomfort have abated, don't assume that further treatment is unnecessary. X-ray photographs must be taken because of the possibility of a fracture. If an ankle sprain is not given proper medical attention, the ankle might be reinjured again and again. Repeat sprains are common on such a traumatized site. That's because a sprained ankle involves torn ligaments, which even with the best medical attention must have time to heal. Be aware, therefore, that emergency care alone is not enough to ensure proper healing of the foot or to prevent future sprains. Emergency treatment is merely first aid, only a stopgag means of allowing ambulation so that you can take yourself to a health professional who is fully skilled in the procedures that will prevent the condition from becoming chronic.

PODIATRIC ATTENTION FOR ACUTE ANKLE SPRAIN

A foot doctor will treat your ankle sprain by first taking an X-ray to determine whether there has been any fracture of the bone where the ligaments are attached. If there has been such a fracture, the doctor will immobilize the ankle in a plaster cast. If no fracture exists, he or she will most likely inject a local anesthetic into the ankle to reduce the pain to a more comfortable level.

The podiatrist might also spray your ankle with ethyl chloride liquid, which will give a momentary sensation of coldness and temporarily allay the pain. The spray will also blanch the skin. After the spray, which acts much like the cold or warm applications used in emergency self-treatment, the blood will surge back into the blanched area as inflammation returns suddenly to the site.

Foot specialists also employ various methods of physical therapy to help restore proper function to the injured ankle. These therapies are the same ones used to relieve the pain of weak arches: ultrasound waves, whirlpool baths, galvanism, diathermy, paraffin baths, and gentle massage.

CAUSE AND CARE OF THE CHRONIC ANKLE SPRAIN

A chronic ankle sprain usually indicates that an acute sprain has been given inadequate or improper attention. The ankle sprains again and again because the ligaments have never healed completely. Muscle development on such a foot is poor, and the foot is weakened. The weakness of the ligaments produces a feeling of instability, and the patient often fears his foot might give way beneath him.

Since the original sprain could have resulted from the foot's being badly positioned when weight was placed on it, the manner in which you walk might need correction. You might even require a corrective shoe to enable you to walk with a normal gait. The feet would then be so placed with each step that no sprain would likely occur. The foot specialist might also prescribe a foot balancer, which is an appliance (such as an orthotic) worn inside the shoe to take the stress off the injured side of the ankle and redistribute the body's weight.

A sprained ankle that feels like a minor injury is not always so minor. Neither is a simple "turned ankle" always simple. The foot being a complex structure, you should not disregard such an injury, for it might be the first of continual minor sprains that will result in a chronically sprained ankle. In fact, sprains that follow an initial sprain can damage the foot severely. An ankle that has been sprained repeatedly might even swell with changes in the weather. You must have a sprained ankle treated promptly and properly to enjoy full mobility.

To care for a chronically sprained ankle, one should regularly perform any exercise that the foot doctor might advise for strengthening the ligaments of the foot. However, if the ligaments that run from side to side in the foot have been stretched by repeated sprains, then you might need to call upon an osteopathic physician or an orthopedic surgeon to receive corrective treatment.

CORRECTING CHRONIC JOINT PAIN

Complete correction of the chronically sprained ankle or other chronic joint pain is available in the form of a well-established injection procedure known as reconstructive therapy, long approved by the American Medical Association and recently adapted for ankle sprains. The technique reconditions a joint into such good repair that it's as if the injury never happened.

Reconstructive therapy involves the injection of a derivative of pharmaceutical-grade cod-liver oil. The derivative, called sodium morrhuate, is combined in a syringe with procaine, an anesthetic. The syringe needle—in this case, about as long and slender as an acupuncture tool—is used to place the stimulating solution in exactly the right place in the ligamentous attachments of the affected joint. In two or three minutes, the anesthetic agent brings relief of pain. The sodium morrhuate then slowly begins the process of repair. It acts as an irritant, causing the body to grow fibrous cells so that torn ligaments and tendons proliferate with new substance. Each treatment causes connective tissue to add on, strengthening formerly unstable joints. Depending on the severity, location, and duration of the disability, the number of injections of reconstructive therapy required varies from one to twenty (and occasionally more).

Developed in the United States, reconstructive therapy has been administered in medicine since 1925. About one million Americans have undergone the treatment. Yet, it remains untaught to most health professionals and goes largely unreported in the medical literature. Mostly, osteopathic physicians—about 150 in the United States and Canada—are the clinicians who enthusiastically administer reconstructive therapy. They use it as an adjunct to manipulation, but the technique is an excellent way to eliminate chronic joint pain and therefore has value in its own right.

FOOT FACT

When tennis players come down to earth after jumping eighteen inches to hit an overhead smash, they exert a force equal to about four times their body weight.

Part Four

Foot Care In Unusual Circumstances

17. *Occupational Difficulties*

THE kind of work you do has long been recognized as a factor in causing health problems. Even the way in which you do your job can cause trouble for individual parts of your body. For example, if you fail to wear safety goggles while working at a grindstone, then sooner or later your eyes might be struck and injured by particles that fly up and away from the rotating wheel.

The feet, too, are exposed to hazards that can cause pain and serious discomfort. Occupational hazards can retard you from satisfying your employer's expectations and therefore can affect your ability to earn a living.

Occupational foot problems can be avoided in most cases, for they are generally caused by the victim. By exercising care, you can prevent them from becoming serious or from arising in the first place. "Caution" is the key word in characterizing the means of avoiding occupational foot difficulties.

Certain foot problems are closely associated with specific occupations. Most of them involve use of the feet as an integral part of accomplishing a piece of work. For instance, before electrical power was used to move the needle on a sewing machine, foot power was used. The operator sometimes developed awful shin splints from constantly manipulating a leg to move the sewing machine's foot treadle. Muscles on the front of the leg would go into spasm, causing the laborer to stop working. Other occupations cause lower-limb difficulties, as well. Today's best-known occupational foot problems are dancer's foot, policeman's heel, march (or soldier's) foot, and waiter's toe.

DANCER'S FOOT

Dancer's foot is a condition that, as you would suspect, chiefly affects those who dance professionally. It is an inflammation, and in severe cases a displacement or fracture, of the two small sesamoid bones beneath the head of the first metatarsal. The sesamoid bones are in the tendons that run beneath the metatarsal to the big toe. (See Figure 17.1.) Their function is to lessen friction as the foot tendons move.

Unusual stresses can injure the two small bones even under the best of circumstances, but they are more susceptible to injury when you are dancing and centering your weight on the balls of the feet. That position permits the easy grace and fluid motion that we associate with dancing, but it places an unusual weight on the sesamoid bones. Damage does not result from such stress alone; it occurs when the stress combines with pressure from the dancer's wearing shoes that are too narrow.

The typical dancing shoe or slipper is narrower than the dancer's foot. It squeezes the foot and exerts added pressure on the sesamoid bones. Inflammation develops in the soft parts of the foot—the tendons, fat, and skin that surround the sesamoid bones. As those soft parts enlarge, they become painful. Later, if abuse continues, the inflammation penetrates deeper into the foot and reaches the bones.

The inflammation and pain jeopardize the dancer's ability to perform. Should he or she ignore the pain, the small, tender, sesamoid bones can fracture or be displaced.

TREATMENT FOR DANCER'S FOOT

Once the dancer recognizes that this foot pain is occupation related and will not disappear by itself, the dancer should seek the help of a

Figure 17.1
The pain of dancer's foot affects the area shaded in this drawing. Notice the sesamoid bones under the head of the first metatarsal at the big toe joint.

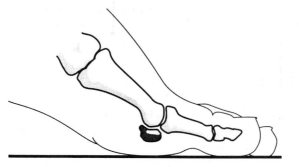

sympathetic foot specialist—immediately. Yet it is not always easy for the sufferer to understand or recognize the nature of the problem. One is inclined to hope that nothing is really wrong. The course of the pain encourages that attitude, for when the dancing begins, the pain begins, and when the performance stops, the pain stops. Furthermore, the pain and inflammation are alleviated by rest—although rest alone will not solve the irritating problem permanently. Professional aid must be sought.

The first thing a podiatrist should do in treating a diagnosed case of dancer's foot is to advise wearing a wider shoe, one that will allow the sole of the foot to expand to its full weight-bearing width. Each part of the foot would then bear its full share of the body's weight.

A felt pad strategically placed in the shoe to fit between the big toe and the first metatarsal will also help. This pad should be thick enough to support the first metatarsal and to lift the weight from the head of the joint. The pad, in effect, carries the weight of the body and relieves pressure from the involved bones.

The methods of physical therapy available to the podiatrist to treat the inflammation and the pain include diathermy and ultrasound. The diathermy treatment, especially, can be used to bake the inflamed area.

FOOT FACT

During his or her life, the average person will walk more than 250,000 miles—the distance from the Earth to the moon.

POLICEMAN'S HEEL

Despite its name, policeman's heel is not a foot condition peculiar to policemen. It is an ailment caused by standing for long periods of time on such inelastic surfaces as concrete or stone. Policemen, especially traffic officers, are susceptible to policeman's heel, it is true; but letter carriers, street cleaners, assembly-line workers, waiters, and many other persons who stand or walk at their work also suffer from the condition.

Policeman's heel, known technically as calcaneal bursitis, is an inflammation of a bursa just under the weight-bearing surfaces of the heel bone. Because of its location, a calcaneal bursitis is painful only when one is standing or walking. It is sharply circumscribed. If one presses a finger into the painful area—no larger than a dime—the bursa will feel much like a large, flattened, spongy pea.

Because the pain from the bursitis arises at the same place as the pain caused by a heel spur, there is a chance that one might be mistaken for the other. The trained foot doctor, however, easily identifies either condition from an X-ray photograph of the heel; if the pain is caused by a bursitis, the photograph will not show the distinctive protruding ridge that is the sign of a calcaneal spur.

Although the problems are distinct from each other, calcaneal spur and calcaneal bursitis are similar in some ways. At first, they can even be treated similarly. As in treatment of heel spurs, the bursitis is relieved by shifting weight away from the point of the inflammation and by easing the pain with physical therapy. Furthermore, they threaten to become quite alike, since continued irritation of the bursitis, if not correctly treated, can lead to the formation of permanent heel spurs. Such permanency is worthwhile to avoid; so our advice is to do everything possible to get rid of policeman's heel.

SELF-TREATMENT FOR POLICEMAN'S HEEL

The first step in treatment of the bursitis is to pad the heel. The procedure is so simple that you can do it at home. Take a felt pad about a quarter-inch thick and two and a half inches square and cut it to the shape of the heel seat in the shoe. Moisten the pad. Then outline the area of pain on your heel with an indelible pencil. To transfer the outline to the pad, step on it with your bare foot. The sketched outline of the bursitis will come off on the moist pad. Next, cut a hole in the pad. The hole should be slightly larger than the outlined area. Then secure the pad permanently in the shoe with a drop of mucilage or glue. When you wear the shoe, the inflamed bursa will float in the hole without touching the adjacent area, and the pressure upon the bursa will be eliminated.

As an adjunct to padding, you can apply heat to the heel with a hot wet cloth or a heating pad. Also good is to soak the foot in a hot solution to take away the inflammation. Prepare the solution by adding two heaping tablespoons of Epsom salts to a gallon of water as hot as comfort allows. Place your foot into the solution and soak for an hour. While you soak, you can read a book, watch television, or perform some other sedentary occupation. As the water cools, add more hot water and continue the soaking. More hot soaks is better than fewer when it comes to ridding yourself of policeman's heel.

PROFESSIONAL TREATMENT FOR POLICEMAN'S HEEL

The practicing podiatrist can carry out those same procedures for you, probably with a greater assurance of success. A foot doctor is able to devise a pad for the foot that's just right. Also, he or she can apply heat to the inflamed bursa with therapy that is more advanced than just hot water or a heating pad. The podiatrist can use ultrasound waves, diathermy, or a whirlpool bath to reduce the inflammation and relieve the acute discomfort.

Chronic cases of calcaneal bursitis might require surgical removal of the bursa. Because the heel is padded with fat, such surgery is somewhat difficult to perform, but it can be accomplished in the doctor's office, without hospitalization. It takes surgical skill. The patient who undergoes such bursal surgery on the heel probably should be immobilized during the several days of recuperation.

Surgery is usually reserved for those cases in which the bursitis does not respond to other treatments.

MARCH (SOLDIER'S) FOOT

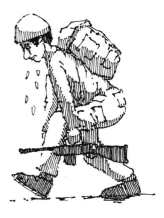

March foot, which was first described medically in 1926, is the spontaneous fracture of one or more metatarsal bones. Because German soldiers who served in World War I were the subjects of the medical study, the condition is sometimes known as soldier's foot or Deutschlander's disease.

March foot is, as the term indicates, an occupational problem of soldiers who are often required to march long distances at a rapid pace with little or no opportunity to rest. The potent combination of extreme fatigue and continued stress can lead eventually to fracture. Soldier's foot was a primary difficulty for fighters in the "war to end all wars."

Civilians seldom suffer from march foot. They rarely march long distances, and those who do march can normally rest at will. They are rarely compelled to continue after becoming aware of strain and fatigue.

As strong as the metatarsal bones are, they can break if one wearily trudges mile after mile. At first, the constant pounding of the march causes only mild swelling and pain—familiar signs to anyone who has ever walked a great distance. For civilians, the signs of danger do not, however, continue beyond the point of discomfort; the warning signs might even disappear altogether. Because of the limited warnings, march foot kind of sneaks up on the civilian. On the other hand, the signs of danger continue for the soldier who is forced to continue to march.

Later, the swelling march foot possibly will occur again and spread slowly along the top of the foot, from the toes toward the ankle. The pain will become severe. Soon, spasm occurs in the muscles between the toes and the metatarsals. Those sudden contractions are similar to and as painful as a charley horse in the calf or thigh muscles. The pain becomes more intense, until it is almost unbearable. Walking becomes almost impossible.

After that point, if one persists in walking or is compelled to march, the metatarsals will break because their muscles cannot support the inflamed bones and arches. Usually, the second or third metatarsal bone breaks, but sometimes both bones fracture.

To treat march foot, one must rest it. Continued foot fatigue must be avoided. In time, the bones will knit and heal. In general, it is neither possible nor necessary to put the foot in a cast. Rather, a podiatrist will place a stiffening appliance, such as a leather or plastic insole, under the foot to hold the bones in place while they heal. Such an appliance is formed to fit the shape of the foot and extends from the webs of the toes (the flesh that holds the toes together) to the back of the heel.

WAITER'S TOE

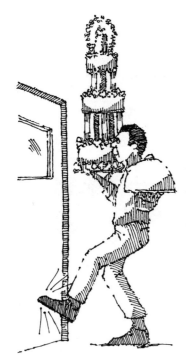

Waiter's toe is a foot problem common among people who attend the dining needs of customers in restaurants. Yet, any individual who abuses his feet as a waiter necessarily does is likely to suffer from waiter's toe.

Kicking a solid object repeatedly will ultimately bring on waiter's toe. A waiter or waitress who is carrying a tray of dishes in both hands often kicks open the kitchen door of the restaurant with his or her foot. If he or she does that continually, day after day, the waiter or waitress will soon suffer the injury that we have designated as waiter's toe.

Although the impact of the door might seem slight, its cumulative effect is sufficient to cause a chronic inflammation at the inner side of the big toe. It can also cause an ingrown toenail, which if ignored can lead to the development of a corn beneath the nail. The pain from all three sources—inflammation, ingrown toenail, and corn beneath the nail—can be intense.

A podiatrist treats waiter's toe in the same manner that he or she treats other toenail problems. The precise procedure for remedying the problem will depend upon its severity and upon the extent of any complications. The only permanent solution to waiter's toe is to refrain from kicking at solid objects, in this instance the swinging door.

Occupational hazards to the feet can be avoided by exercising care. If a trauma to the feet does occur or if the feet begin to hurt and affect your ability to carry out your work, then seek the cause. A health professional might help.

No foot problem should be permitted to interfere with your livelihood. In most instances, by taking some simple precautions you can enjoy complete foot comfort while working at your chosen trade, craft, or profession.

18. *The Perils of Jogging*

PEOPLE often experience a wonderfully elated feeling after engaging in an outdoor run. Running offers many benefits to the body, mind, and emotions. However, unless done along woodland paths or through open fields, running, even slow jogging, can be hazardous to your health—especially if performed on city streets.

Yes, America is on the run. Millions have turned to jogging as the alternative to traditional games and sports. Jogging, an aerobic activity, requires the use of lots of oxygen over a relatively long period so that the circulatory system gets conditioned into shape.

The main difference between jogging and running is speed. Putting one leg in front of the other at a rate of a mile in seven minutes is running. Taking longer than seven minutes to go a mile is jogging. Some people jog at a turtle-like pace, humorously called slogging.

All aerobic exponents—sloggers, joggers, and runners—are after one thing: cardiovascular fitness. The question is whether the benefits of their activity outweigh the risks. Are there dangers connected with jogging?

JOGGING MAY BE HAZARDOUS TO YOUR FOOT HEALTH

The cardiovascular system is an important body structure, but so is the skeletal system. It takes in all the bony parts of the body. If a person ruins his or her ankles, knees, hips, back, or other parts of the skeletal

FOOT FACT

Race walking, then called "pedestrianism," was the biggest spectator sport in the United States at the end of the nineteenth century. The participants wore sturdy leather boots.

system by jogging on a hard surface to enhance the cardiovascular system, what has been gained?

Dr. Gordon Falknor, a Chicago podiatrist, told members attending a 1983 meeting of the Illinois Podiatry Association that he had discovered an ailment he called "jogger's foot." Now, a number of years later, that condition has been affirmed by many other foot doctors as one of the problems they commonly treat.

"The symptoms are similar to trauma and tendinitis of the Achilles tendon just above its attachment to the heel bone," Dr. Falknor explained. He added that tissues of the feet and ankle take a terrific pounding from jogging on concrete or blacktop surfaces, leading to the eventual breakdown of those tissues.

Blisters on the feet are another source of discomfort connected with jogging. Blisters are caused by the friction of the skin's rubbing against an unyielding surface or edge inside the running shoe. A seam, or even a crease or darn in a sock, can cause them, too. Sometimes, blisters are quite unpredictable in occurrence, although usually after the damage is done it is relatively easy to find the cause. The feet can swell during exercise, pushing the skin against irritating seams or surfaces that had seemed quite comfortable before.

Black toenails are a third jogging hazard. They are caused by shoes that do not fit properly; the toe is jammed hard against the roof of the shoe on every step. The toe starts to bleed under the nail, and the blood causes a painful buildup of pressure. The nail might then die, to be replaced slowly by a new growth some weeks later. Meanwhile, the nail is fairly tender.

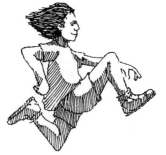

Cramping, a sudden and sustained spasm of a muscle, can be exceedingly painful and unexpected. Medical experts say that cramping in the calf muscles or in the feet themselves has not yet been fully explained in joggers. It's suspected that an imbalance of electrolytes and fluid (often caused by excessive sweating) is one source of the difficulty. Cramping can affect the lower limbs during the closing stages of a jog.

The prolonged, unchanging use of a certain muscle group can also increase the likelihood of cramping. Ironically, a marathon course with one or two hills in the latter stages, where a slightly different running action is used to tackle the incline, might be less likely to cause cramping than would a totally flat, unremitting course with no such contrasts.

Most injuries to joggers occur in the lower leg and foot. Apart from unlucky accidents, such as putting your foot down a hole or treading on a stone, nearly all such injuries are caused by overuse. Repeating the same running action a vast number of times can lead to injury. Often, the Achilles tendon, knee, and shin are involved, along with the foot itself.

The Achilles tendon, which attaches the calf muscles to the heel bone, is the site of a lot of pain for both the beginner and the experienced jogger. In its mildest form, such tendinitis can include some swelling and tenderness to the touch. It can be brought on simply by the beginner's overdoing his exercise with too much jogging in the early stages or by his trying to run on his toes.

SHIN SPLINTS AND STRESS FRACTURES

A shin splint, or shin soreness, consists of a sharp pain and tightness on the outside of the shin. The problem arises because the anterior tibial (shin) muscles, which also support the arch mechanism of the foot, have little room for the expansion they do during sustained exercise. The subsequent buildup of pressure within the restraining sheath restricts blood circulation. Possible causes are a high jogging mileage; shoe soles that do not flex sufficiently; a lack of shock absorption in the heel, allowing shock to be sent through the shin; and an imbalance of strength between shin and calf muscles.

FOOT FACT

Injuries to the foot and knee account for half of all athletic injuries and 70 percent of injuries to runners.

Stress fracture is a common injury among joggers who aren't used to running on pavement. The stress fracture usually occurs in either of the two long bones of the lower leg (tibia and fibula) or in the long, narrow metatarsals of the foot. Symptoms and signs of stress fracture are similar to those for shin soreness. Sometimes, local swelling and tenderness occur just above the ankle, where constant stress across any of the long bones can produce a tiny crack that does not always show up on an X-ray.

Runner's knee, sometimes called *chondromalacia patella*, is believed to be caused by a softening of the cartilage of the undersurface of the kneecap (the patella). The kneecap normally moves over the end of the thigh bone. The softening might be caused by excessive rotation of the knee as the foot hits the ground, possibly due to the athlete's being slightly knock-kneed or bow-legged or having a foot imbalance.

RETROGRESSIVE FORCES CREATE BODY IMBALANCE

George Sheehan, M.D., the medical adviser for *Runner's World* magazine, says, "When you run, three things happen to your body—and two of them are bad."

The only good thing is that you build more stamina for jogging. The first bad item, retrogressive force, creates the second—body imbalance. For instance, the muscles in back of the body—calves, hamstrings, buttocks, and lower back—grow strong and inflexible. Muscles in front

Which Shoe for Which Sport?

Whatever happened to plain old sneakers?

What happened was a phenomenon called the running boom, which in the mid-1970s not only led to the development of technologically superior running shoes, but served as the catalyst for exercise physiologists and foot specialists, who went on to determine that each sport places different stresses on our feet and legs, and often on our entire bodies. The result is that a remarkable selection of biomechanically engineered footwear has become available to meet the needs of each sport.

The plethora of choices is wonderful if you know what you're looking for in athletic shoes but terribly daunting if you don't. For example, how is a beginning fitness walker to know whether the blue shoe with the waffle-patterned sole is correct for his needs? Do running shoes make sense for a volleyball game? Is it wise for a woman to slip into men's tennis shoes and perform her exercises? Are high-top basketball shoes better than low ones?

To find the answers, we spoke with the experts—sports podiatrists. Also, we came upon an excellent booklet put out by the Foot Locker/Lady Foot Locker chain of athletic footwear stores. *How to Choose Athletic Shoes,* written by noted health and medical writer Joan R. Heilman (in consultation with sports podiatrist Lloyd S. Smith and orthopedic surgeon John F. Waller Jr.), provides an education on sports shoes. We were fortunate enough to be given permission to use or adapt some of that booklet's wealth of information here.

Running shoes are designed to move you in one direction only—straight ahead. Their soles curve up in front and back, have a slightly elevated heel with a firm counter (which provides the heel with stiffness), and a sharply bevelled edge for stability. The counter in a better shoe might be reinforced with an external stabilizer and a rigid collar of high-strength plastic between the counter and the cushioned midsole. The nylon uppers are soft, light, and flexible with suede, leather, or pigskin at the stress points. Hard rubber soles may be grooved or studded for traction.

Track shoes require lightness of weight with sprint spikes in the sole. The uppers may be made of nylon reinforced with suede, but there is no padding between your feet and the thin synthetic sole. For distance runners on a track, the spikes are more padded and elevated under the heel. Road racers should wear shoes that have spikeless, flat, rubber outer soles and cushioned midsoles.

Football shoes require thick, full-grain leather for protection from foot abuse. The shoes feature sturdy counters, high or low tops, and spiked rubber soles. If the playing field is naturally hard, then the cleats should be numerous, large, and made of molded rubber. For Astroturf and other hard, artificial surfaces, numerous tiny cleats are required for traction. When playing on soft grass, use replaceable cleats with hard plastic studs.

Soccer shoes require soft, supple, full-grain leather with hard rubber or synthetic cleated soles and a long protective tongue at the instep. For soft playing fields, there should be six replaceable plastic cleats. For hard fields, one-piece bottoms with molded cleats are correct.

Tennis shoes require good lateral support for the rapid moves in many directions. The soles should be flat, hard, square-edged, and have less elevation to the heels. The cushioned midsole absorbs shock, and a firm counter keeps the heel securely in place. The uppers should be made of leather, nylon mesh, or canvas. On clay courts, soft rubber soles with a flat, pilled, or open tread is best for preventing clay clogs. On hard courts, nubbed or patterned polyurethane and rubber soles work well.

Racquetball, squash, and **handball** shoes require tacky rubber soles for traction on slippery wood floors. The thick and flexible soles are rounded along the edges. Inner soles supply good cushioning, and uppers may be of nylon mesh.

Baseball and **softball** shoes require nylon mesh and leather uppers, long tongue flaps to fold down over the laces, and firm synthetic soles with steel spikes, molded plastic cleats, or hard rubber cleats.

Basketball requires heavier-weight footgear with protection for heels and ankles such as is afforded by high-top shoes. Hard rubber-cup soles may be ridged for traction on wood floors. Cushioning should be present at the midsoles and ankles.

Biking shoes require a synthetic or leather sole that is inflexible and uncushioned. Holes should be present in the sole to allow for evaporation of perspiration. Some biking shoes lock into the pedal assembly to minimize foot motion. Non-competitive riders may look for more conventional shoes of composition or rubber soles with grooves or bars that help the feet grip the pedals.

Volleyball requires high-top or low-top shoes with mesh and leather uppers and reinforced toes. Midsoles should be well cushioned under the metatarsals. Soles may be composed of ridged-gum crepe or rubber compounds for good traction on wood.

Aerobic workout shoes require raised heels, firm counters, wrapped soft rubber soles, and good shock absorbability. Made of soft garment leather, canvas, or nylon, they look ungainly because of added comfort features.

Fitness walking shoes require nylon mesh or leather uppers and strong counters—and, occasionally, devices to restrict lateral movement. There should be cushioning under the toes, plus slightly elevated heels for forward thrusting. The soles should be made of rubber or composition materials.

of the body—shins, quadriceps, and abdomen—fail to keep pace. A strength imbalance develops.

As one becomes a better runner, the tightness and imbalance increase—and so do the chances for knee pain, shin splints, Achilles tendinitis, pulls of the calf or hamstring muscles, and irritation of the sciatic nerve. Reported most commonly among joggers, however, are foot disorders.

Foot ligaments exposed to stresses and strains elongate and undergo inflammatory changes that cause discomfort. If the jogging continues even in the face of the suffering, the ligaments elongate further and degenerate, losing their supportive function and permitting excessive motion of the joints. Excessive play and misalignment of the many joints will inflame the surrounding capsules and foot surfaces. Joint inflammation becomes the source of arthritic pain. Over time, surgery on those capsules might become necessary.

If the stress of jogging continues, irritation to the foot joints is inevitable, structural damage to the joint surfaces must occur, and degenerative arthritis sets in. Nature tends to respond to those chronic insults by attempting to reconstruct the joints or by forming a bulwark against the irritation with an overgrowth of bone that will often result in a deformed joint (called an arthrosis) or a bony spur (as on the heel bone). If changes are recognized early enough, the cycle of damage is reversible; but if the changes proceed too far, the bony growth becomes well-established and the joint might get beyond repair.

THREE FOOT TYPES SUFFER MOST FROM JOGGING

Retrogressive forces from jogging are most apt to occur in the three dysfunctional foot types: long first toe; Morton's syndrome foot (long second toe, short first toe); and outwardly splayed metatarsals.

Jogging puts those three types of feet through a sequence of pathological events that might bring on permanent injury. Here, perhaps for the first time anywhere, is a blow-by-blow account that shows anatomically fluent readers how jogging can affect the foot:

1. The first metatarsal bone separates from the second metatarsal, causing the first bone to angle from the midline of the foot.
2. The big toe turns abruptly at an opposite angle to the midline and creates a protruding, angulated bunion.
3. The final phases of walking cause a pulling of the muscles on the inner side of the foot and act excessively on the big toe between the first and second metatarsal.
4. The gap between the first and second metatarsal grows progressively wider.

FOOT FACT

Runners who cover more than fifty miles a week develop feet that are longer and flatter than those of their lower-mileage colleagues.

5. More forces of retrogression cause the second, third, fourth, and fifth toes to contract.
6. A bending upward of the toe bones in the lesser digits sets in.
7. Calluses tend to form at the tips of the toes and on the tops of the bent joints because of pressure against the shoes.
8. The back parts of the toe bones drop down.
9. The capsules and tendons on the bent toe-bottom surfaces become contracted while those on the top stretch.
10. Pressure and imbalance affect the second, third, fourth, and fifth metatarsal bones, which are forced back to exert pressure against the center of the foot.
11. The ball of the foot depresses downward to the ground.
12. Calluses form on the plantar skin, and muscular cramps develop throughout the tiny foot muscles.
13. Muscle spasms and weakening ligaments permit all the bones in the rear of the foot to sag.
14. The heel bone turns downward on the inner side, and its front portion depresses.
15. The ankle pronates (turns inward).
16. A reverse process of torque throws the entire foot out of balance.
17. The downward position of the heel places extra stress upon the front of the foot, which responds by turning outward, away from the body's midline.
18. The entire foot now bears weight on its inner border to force it into more pronation, thus placing strain on the medial angle ligaments and upon the tendon of the calf muscles.
19. The Achilles tendon deviates to the outside and shortens.
20. Constant pulling at the tendon attachment on the back of the heel bone causes extra calcium to accumulate with arthritic spurring.
21. The shortened tendon places more strain throughout the front segments of the foot so that any protective muscular action is overwhelmed.
22. Stress continues from the retrogressive forces and is imparted further upon the ligaments, then upon the joint capsules, and ultimately upon the joints themselves.
23. Joints so strained separate slightly, and the foot undergoes a functional deformity.
24. Persistence of the stress ultimately converts the functional deformity into a structural one.
25. The foot problem becomes permanent, with surgery usually the only sufficient way to correct it.

FOOT FACT

Computers the size of small, thin wristwatches are built into some of the newest high-technology athletic shoes. These devices can register average speed, stride length, distance covered, trip time, and even calories burned.

HEEL CUSHION CORRECTS JOGGING'S JOLTING EFFECTS

A fairly new correction for the jolting effects of jogging has come on the market. Sofstride heel cushions accommodate the feet and do away with the injurious effects arising from fast ambulation on the flat, hard, unyielding surfaces so consistent with running, jogging, or slogging. Sofstrides reduce shock that strikes the bones and soft tissues and effectively ward off shin splints.

Sofstrides are cushioning devices made of Kraton rubber, a synthetic compound. Light in weight, they cup the heels with pleasant softness. The heel cushion is worn against the bare skin inside the hosiery. Thus, the heel bones are protected from overly sharp collisions with the shoe insole and, subsequently, the ground. Furthermore, body load gets dispersed by Sofstrides across both feet evenly and is not focused on any areas of foot weakness.

FOOT FACT

To make one athletic shoe, fifteen to twenty-four separate pieces are assembled.

JOGGING IS NOT FOR EVERYONE

Bernard L. Gladieux Jr., former editor of *The Jogger*, the monthly newsletter of the National Jogging Association, says, "If you are over thirty, you should check with your doctor before you begin any exercise program. If you're over forty, take a treadmill stress test to make sure you're in shape."

Since jogging can be hazardous to your health, especially your foot health, take note of this sage advice: Don't run out on your feet, for jogging or running brings on foot problems.

19. *Foot Care for Diabetics*

HEALTHY skin is actually a protective envelope against many disease-causing organisms. But if the skin dries and thickens, it becomes brittle, cracks, and develops fissures that might permit bacteria to infect the body. That is also true if the skin is cut, abraded, scratched, or ruptured in any other manner.

Normally, the body can successfully fight off an invasion of pathogenic organisms. Once the skin has been broken, white blood cells, antibodies, and other components of the immune system mobilize to repel the invaders. Thus, although a break in normal, healthy skin can be painful or uncomfortable, it is generally of minor consequence. A local sore might develop, but it will heal quickly.

In contrast, the skin of the diabetic isn't normal. Its effectiveness in defending the body against infection and disease is reduced, and the tissues beneath the skin are poorly prepared to fight the invading organisms. A cut or sore on the foot of a diabetic might develop into an ulcer or gangrene, either of which poses a serious medical problem.

Diabetes, of course, is not a disease of the feet; but the importance of proper foot care for diabetics is widely recognized. Diabetes, a chronic disorder in which the body has difficulty absorbing carbohydrates, is caused by a lack of sufficient insulin, a hormone produced in the pancreas. Body cells need insulin to metabolize carbohydrates; if insulin is lacking, the glucose that would normally be used by the cells is instead excreted in urine or perspiration. Sugar-laden perspiration constitutes a perfect medium for the growth of fungi that can infect the feet.

Diabetes can also impair the circulation of the blood, and poor circulation makes it difficult for the body to repair quickly the physical damage from a cut or sore.

A general systemic disease, diabetes requires continual medical care. Part of that care must be directed to the feet, which are extremely vulnerable to infection. Any foot infection, although of minor significance to most people, can become a matter of life or death to a diabetic. Therefore, the diabetic should visit a foot doctor every month. The podiatrist, by performing tasks that a diabetic dare not do for himself without endangering his health, aids the physician in managing the disease. Proper foot care can help the diabetic live a more normal, healthier, and happier life.

ATHLETE'S FOOT AND THE DIABETIC

The skin of a diabetic's foot presents a perfect medium for the infection of athlete's foot. The foot perspires excessively; the thin, tender skin becomes soggy; and resistance to the fungus infection is lowered. For protection, the person with diabetes should bathe his or her feet daily in warm soapy water, then dry thoroughly between the toes and rub the feet with alcohol. To absorb accumulating perspiration, a foot powder may be used. Cotton or wool socks or stockings—never non-absorbent nylon ones—and well-ventilated shoes should be worn.

Athlete's foot must always be treated promptly and thoroughly; but in the case of the diabetic, strong fungicidal agents containing caustic drugs must not be applied, for they can injure the skin. The consulted doctor will recommend mild anti-fungal creams, ointments, or powders. Of particular merit for the diabetic is griseofulvin, the anti-fungal antibiotic administered in pill form. It reduces chronic fungus infections, is an excellent treatment against athlete's foot, and does not produce any harsh local reactions.

CALLUSES AND CORNS

Diabetics are prone to callus formation, a source of danger. The thickening and enlarging of callused skin can cause the flesh beneath to "liquify"—that is, the cells in the papillary layer of the skin disintegrate. Infection and ulceration can follow. Should even a painless abscess form and not be opened and drained, infection can spread into the surrounding area.

A callus cannot stretch when weight is placed upon it. Such inelastic skin might crack or split and open the body to a bacterial invasion. To maintain the elasticity and flexibility of the skin, the thickness of the callus should be reduced, carefully.

When the callus is small, the diabetic patient can pare it with a fine emery board or with a pumice stone. Larger, thicker calluses must be trimmed with proper instruments by a health professional who does that work as part of his or her daily routine. A podiatrist who treats calluses must take a more rigid, thoroughly careful approach when the patient is a diabetic, because the skin must not be broken in any way.

Corns are also a problem for the person with diabetes. A corn, like a callus, can ulcerate, which is always serious for a diabetic.

"Bathroom surgery" must not be attempted. Anyone who has a corn might be tempted toward self-treatment, but cutting the corn could be limb-threatening for the diabetic. (See Figure 19.1.) The core of the corn must be removed to bring relief from the discomfort, but if it is taken out incorrectly, an ulcer can form. The diabetic should never attempt to remove the central corn portion. That task must be left to a doctor who knows how to take it out without causing bleeding.

Diabetics who develop corns should consult a podiatrist at regular intervals for corn removal and toe padding with protective felt. Diabetics should never treat their corns with any strong cauterizing agents. They must especially beware of commercial corn remedies that could cause serious chemical burns.

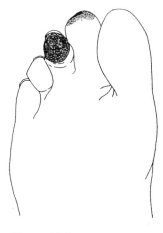

Figure 19.1
People who suffer from diabetes can cause themselves real harm by self-administering to painful corns. In this artist's rendering, a diabetic has developed gangrene at the ends of the second and third toe because of home care given to the right foot.

CUTS AND SCRATCHES

Any injury to the skin on a diabetic's foot—a cut, scratch, sore, or burn—needs to be attended to quickly. Wash those lesions with soap and water to remove all foreign matter, then cover with a protective sterile dressing. Regular adhesive tape must not be used to hold the dressing in place; it would weaken diabetic skin even further. Instead, the dressing should be affixed with masking tape, hypoallergenic medical tape, transparent tape (such as Scotch), or gauze roller bandages (long rolls of fine-mesh gauze in bandage form).

INGROWN TOENAILS

Ingrown toenails are to be feared in particular by diabetics because of the danger that an infection will become gangrenous. For that reason, diabetics must exercise great care when clipping their toenails and must file them smooth. Jagged nails can be snagged by objects and ripped. Diabetics can also help prevent ingrown nails by wearing properly fitted shoes that in no way impinge on the toes. Molded shoes are recommended.

If an ingrown nail does develop, then the infection must be localized and cured at once. To prevent an infection from spreading, the foot surgeon will excise the portion of the nail that is pressing into the infected area and will drain all pockets of pus. The podiatrist will continue to treat the nail until all danger from the infection is removed.

Proper foot care is important to everyone, but to the diabetic it is doubly important; problems that are minor in a healthy person can become major in a diabetic. Thus, the diabetic must diligently observe the rules for proper foot care if he wishes to avoid complications that can seriously damage his health or even imperil his life.

20. *Foot Care During Pregnancy*

NATURE helps prepare every pregnant woman for the demands of childbearing, and if the woman regularly visits a physician and follows sound medical advice on what to do about her nutrition and exercise, then she should have a comfortable pregnancy. Because the mother-to-be is often advised to walk for exercise, she should give special attention to the shoes she wears as well as to her foot health in general.

The body carries an additional weight as the fetus develops. If the figure is to be held erect, a special effort must be made to maintain good posture. The woman who carries herself well during this period is not merely admired by others; her spirits seem improved, and her body feels as if it functions better. Furthermore, since the uterus (womb) is subject to gravitational pull, poor carriage might cause unnecessary strain, which conceivably could bring on complications.

The shoes the pregnant woman wears must be appropriate and fitted with care, for during these months her feet carry a greater than normal burden. Therefore, pregnancy is no time for wearing pointed-toe or high-heeled shoes. Nor is it a time for the loose, casual, flat shoes that the mother-to-be may always have enjoyed wearing at home. The proper pair of shoes for her are low-heeled, rubber- or leather-soled, six-eyelet oxfords. The shoes' uppers should be made of a strong fabric or of leather, and the heels should be less than an inch and a half in height. Those shoes might not be fashionable, but they are the most healthful to wear during pregnancy.

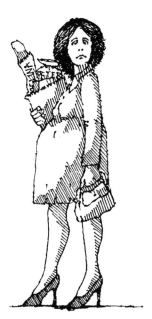

Pregnancy is no time for wearing pointed-toe or high-heeled shoes.

149

Great Daily Exercises

Walking is by far the best general exercise, but you must walk correctly. To do so, set your feet straight ahead. Your body weight will be transmitted directly through the ankle joints and be distributed evenly over the feet. Then, with head erect, shoulders squared, and weight evenly balanced, stride forward.

Although walking is the best general exercise for the feet, it will not always stretch cramped foot muscles. For a quick pickup after a hard or tiring day, plunge your feet into warm water, then splash them with cold water, and then towel briskly.

Walking, daily care, and specific exercise of the lower limbs will lead to healthier feet. You can exercise the small muscles of the foot by walking barefoot on soft surfaces such as sand, a lawn, or a deep pile rug. Also, it strengthens your foot muscles if, at various intervals during the day, you walk on your toes or stand on one foot and swing the other back and forth.

Performing the following illustrated exercises will tone up your foot muscles:

Exercise 1.   To stretch the tendons on the top of the foot, sit in a relaxed position, bare feet on the floor, and try to pick up a Turkish towel, marbles, or a pencil with your toes.

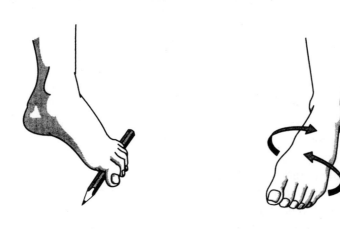

Exercise 1   Exercise 2

Exercise 2.   To relieve stiffness of the ankle joint, sit in a chair, cross one leg over the other, and bend your top foot down and then up; rotate your foot in one direction and then in the other; repeat ten or fifteen times. Then cross your other leg and exercise your other foot.

Exercise 3. To relieve rigidity in the ankle and longitudinal arch, alternately stand flat on your feet and rise to your toes. Do this several times.

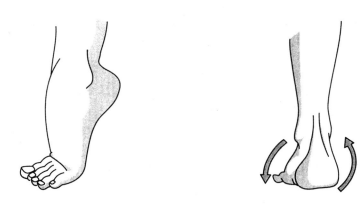

Exercise 3   Exercise 4

Exercise 4. To relieve strain on the two inner longitudinal arches, roll your feet outward fifteen or twenty times so that your weight rests on the outer borders of your feet.

Exercise 5. To strengthen toe muscles, stand with your feet parallel and bend your toes up as far as you can.

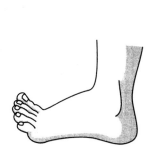
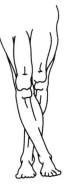

Exercise 5   Exercise 6

Exercise 6. To bring into use every muscle of balance, stand with knees stiff and legs crossed – like a scissors – and feet parallel and slightly apart so that the weight of your body is distributed evenly over both feet. Hold this cross-legged position for a minute or two; reverse.

Exercise 7. To strengthen calf and heel muscles, sit on the floor with your legs straight ahead and bend your feet upward as far as possible.

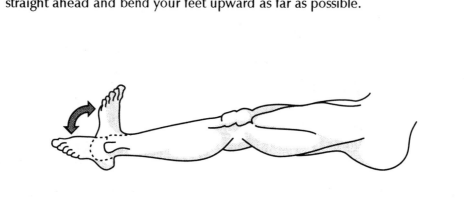

Exercise 7

Exercise 8. To strengthen arches and tone up calves, sit with your legs straight ahead and turn the soles of your feet closely together.

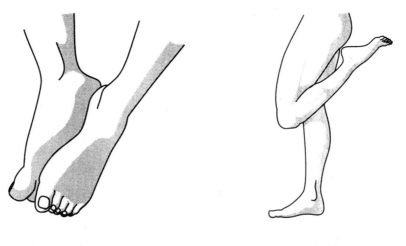

Exercise 8   Exercise 9

Exercise 9. To exercise thigh muscles, lean forward against a wall so that your weight is on your arms, and then kick your buttocks with the back of each foot.

Fitting such shoes poses only a minor problem. Because the feet expand during the day, the shoes should be fitted in the late afternoon or evening, when the feet are close to their maximum length.

As the fetus grows, the feet of the pregnant woman will carry an increasing weight and will spread in both length and width. Therefore, it is wise to own a pair of supportive shoes one size larger and wider than ordinarily required. To ensure that one pair will fit throughout the entire pregnancy, the expectant woman might have her shoes fitted with an extra insole when she buys them. Then, as her feet expand, she can remove the insole to enlarge the shoe. Of course, anyone who can afford to buy new shoes every few weeks during her pregnancy can be always assured of having properly fitted shoes.

In any case, the pregnant woman should not wear her usual footwear—unless she ordinarily wears low-heeled, sensible, rubber-soled, oxford-type shoes. Just as maternity clothes are necessary, so are "maternity shoes" required—if a woman is to enjoy complete foot health through her nine months of pregnancy.

Special care should also be given to the feet. Any unusual growths deserve immediate attention. Corns, calluses, warts, and ingrown toenails should be removed as soon as possible, no matter where they occur on the foot. That will eliminate foot pain or fatigue and thus decrease the possibility that an unusual gait or stance will exert strain on the muscles, ligaments, and bones.

From time to time, the legs should be examined for varicose veins. The appearance of such veins might indicate a circulatory problem. In any case, if the red net-like veins appear, then the woman should provide foot and leg support by wearing strong elastic stockings of narrow mesh.

FOOT FACT

Only 11 percent of the people who buy tennis shoes wear them to play tennis; just 18 percent of running-shoe purchasers buy them for running.

RULES FOR FOOT HEALTH DURING PREGNANCY

To enjoy good foot health during pregnancy, observe several simple pregnancy-related rules in conjunction with the rules for general foot health (given in the "Basic Foot Care" chapter). Some of those general rules deserve repetition. One should, of course, keep the feet clean. The hygiene-conscious expectant woman will habitually wash her feet at least once a day. Powders and lubricating creams may be used regularly. Finally, the toenails must be clipped carefully in the prescribed straight-across manner.

Other rules, already noted, for foot health during pregnancy:

- Wear larger shoes as your feet enlarge during pregnancy.
- If you buy larger shoes to be worn during pregnancy, then do so in the late afternoon or evening.

- Do not wear high-heeled shoes, but do wear comfortable, low-heeled shoes.
- Give immediate attention to any foot problem that arises.

The same way you go to the dentist for preventive checkups, visit a podiatrist for foot maintenance at least once during the prenatal period.

Proper care of the feet is a small part of the total physical care during pregnancy. It is, however, extremely important, because the health of the feet can affect the posture. The body might compensate for weak, painful, unbalanced feet with strains and stresses on other parts of the body; such accommodations can be harmful. The wisest course is to take proper care of the feet.

FOOT EXERCISE

To continue to enjoy good foot health, you should exercise the muscles of the feet. The exercises given elsewhere in this chapter are as beneficial during pregnancy as at any other time. Pregnancy will not prevent you from doing those simple exercises daily; they should take no more than five minutes.

About the Authors

DONALD S. PRITT, doctor of podiatric medicine, has practiced in West Virginia and Ohio for thirty-one years. An active member of the Academy of Ambulatory Foot Surgeons, Dr. Pritt has had more than one hundred of his original research papers published in medical journals. The professional magazine received by every podiatrist in the country, *Journal of Current Podiatric Medicine*, awarded Dr. Pritt the annual Maxwell N. Cupshan Memorial Award for professional excellence in the years 1975, 1976, 1978, 1981, and 1989.

He is a graduate of the Illinois College of Podiatric Medicine and a former trustee of the New York College of Podiatric Medicine. Dr. Pritt's specialty is ambulatory foot surgery, but he also holds patents for running shoes, heel shock absorbers, and other products.

MORTON WALKER, doctor of podiatric medicine, left almost seventeen years of practice in 1969 to work full time as a free-lance medical journalist. The author of fifty books and nearly 1,400 magazine, newspaper, and clinical journal articles, Dr. Walker has won twenty-two medical journalism awards, including two Jesse H. Neal Editorial Achievement Awards from the American Business Press. Ten times has Dr. Walker won either the American Podiatry Association's William J. Stickel Annual Award for Research and Writing or its Annual Hall of Science Award for Scientific Exhibits. He won both the coveted Gold Medal and the Silver Medal from the American Podiatry Association in 1964. Dr. Walker has won the Maxwell N. Cupshan Memorial Award eleven times.

His special areas of interest are holistic medicine, orthomolecular nutrition, and safe, non-toxic, alternative methods of healing diseases, dysfunctions, and disorders.

Index